Value-Based Approaches
to Spine Care

Rajiv K. Sethi • Anna K. Wright
Michael G. Vitale

Editors

Value-Based Approaches to Spine Care

Sustainable Practices in an Era of Over-Utilization

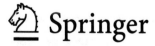 Springer

Editors
Rajiv K. Sethi, MD
Neuroscience Institute
Virginia Mason Medical Center
Seattle, WA
USA

Anna K. Wright, PhD
Neuroscience Institute
Virginia Mason Medical Center
Seattle, WA
USA

Michael G. Vitale, MD, MPH
Columbia University
New York, NY
USA

ISBN 978-3-030-31945-8   ISBN 978-3-030-31946-5   (eBook)
https://doi.org/10.1007/978-3-030-31946-5

This Springer imprint is published by the registered company Springer Nature Switzerland AG
The registered company address is: Gewerbestrasse 11, 6330 Cham, Switzerland

Preface

As our society moves from volume to value in the treatment of spinal disorders, we will be increasingly faced with the challenge to move away from yester-care where fee for service healthcare has demanded large volumes of spinal procedures. The aim of this text is to gather thought leaders and provide an up-to-date synopsis of efforts to enhance value in the care of spinal conditions.

The first portion of this book will describe the macro issues around value-based healthcare initiatives that bring together the principles of health economics along with the topic of utilization of spinal procedures. While there is no standard for utilization of any given procedure, we are clearly seeing an upward trend in the United States coupled with increasing costs and stagnant outcomes in certain procedures. In others, such as the treatment of adult spinal deformity, we are seeing a group of patients who can show dramatic improvement in quality of life with successful surgery. At the same time, many centers experience high complication rates and significant morbidity and mortality in patients who have not undergone risk stratification and optimization of those factors that can be improved. The Seattle Spine Team approach is published in peer review as the first value-based paradigm to improve short-term complication rates in the treatment of some of the most complex spinal conditions from a multidisciplinary perspective. This approach was later applied to all patients receiving elective lumbar fusion. This work has led to selective referrals from all regions of the United States by private payors where patients are flown to Seattle for spinal specialty care. Private payors are no longer willing to allow the fee for service principles of yester-care to dominate their own healthcare arena.

The main sections of this book describe specific efforts to enhance value in an era of overutilization of spinal procedures in the United States. Some of this will involve collaboration with registries, and we have asked our Dutch colleagues in Nijmegen for their expertise. We have also looked at technology and how this will help us in the future as we move to more value-based paradigms. The reader will also understand the essence of a multidisciplinary spine model as the answer to many of our current conundrums.

I would like to thank my coeditors, Anna K. Wright, PhD, and Michael G. Vitale, MD, for their collaboration and expertise in forming this book. They have both been essential players in the field of spine safety and value, and I am grateful to them for their camaraderie and team spirit. Michael G. Vitale, MD, has been my brother in the spine safety movement for many years, and my admiration for him continues to grow. I dedicate this book to my mother and father (Brahm and Chander), my wife (Aya), and my four kids (Ariya, Suriya, Anika, and Karina). Particularly, this book is meant to highlight principles that will make spinal care sustainable for the next generation who will undoubtedly need access to high-quality surgeons and teams. As an American patriot and spinal surgeon, I worry that this access will suffer in an era where the costs are growing out of proportion to GDP growth. We must do everything possible to improve our industry for the benefit of our children and generations to come.

Seattle, WA, USA   Rajiv K. Sethi, MD

Contents

Contributors

Michael A. Bohl, MD Department of Neurosurgery, Barrow Neurological Institute, St. Joseph's Hospital and Medical Center, Phoenix, AZ, USA

Douglas C. Burton, MD Department of Orthopaedic Surgery, Kansas City Medical Center, Kansas City, KS, USA

Marinus De Kleuver, MD Department of Orthopaedic Surgery, Radboud University Nijmegen Medical Center, Nijmegen, The Netherlands

Sayf S. A. Faraj, MD Department of Orthopaedic, Radboud University Medical Center, Nijmegen, The Netherlands

Daniel J. Finch, BA Department of Orthopaedic, University of Utah, Salt Lake City, UT, USA

Tufts University, Boston, MA, USA

Andrew S. Friedman, MD Neuroscience Institute, Virginia Mason Medical Center, Seattle, WA, USA

Department of Physical Medicine and Rehabilitation, Virginia Mason Medical Center, Seattle, WA, USA

Andrew I. Gitkind, MD Division of Interventional Spine, Department of Rehabilitation Medicine, Montefiore Medical Center, Albert Einstein College of Medicine, The Bronx, NY, USA

Tsjitske M. Haanstra, PhD Department of Orthopaedic, Radboud University Medical Center, Nijmegen, The Netherlands

Gary S. Kaplan, MD Virginia Mason Medical Center, Seattle, WA, USA

Han Jo Kim, MD Department of Orthopaedic, Hospital for Special Surgery, New York, NY, USA

Jean-Christophe A. Leveque, MD Neuroscience Institute, Virginia Mason Medical Center, Seattle, WA, USA

Department of Neurosurgery, Virginia Mason Medical Center, Seattle, WA, USA

Brook I. Martin, PhD, MPH Department of Orthopaedic, University of Utah, Salt Lake City, UT, USA

Robert S. Mecklenburg, MD Center for Healthcare Solutions, Department of Medicine, Virginia Mason Hospital and Seattle Medical Center, Seattle, WA, USA

Richard Menger, MD Department of Neurosurgery, New York-Presbyterian Hospital-Columbia and Cornell, New York, NY, USA

Sohail K. Mirza, MD, MPH Department of Orthopaedic, Dartmouth-Hitchcock Medical Center, Lebanon, NH, USA

Stephen L. Ondra, MD North Star Healthcare Consulting, LLC, Williston, FL, USA

Rajiv K. Sethi, MD Neuroscience Institute, Departments of Neurosurgery Health Services, Virginia Mason Medical Center, Seattle, WA, USA

Miranda L. van Hooff, MD Department of Orthopaedic Surgery, Radboud University Medical Center, Nijmegen, The Netherlands

Michael G. Vitale, MD, MPH Pediatric Spine and Scoliosis Service, Division of Pediatric Orthopaedic, Quality & Strategy, Orthopaedic Surgery, Columbia University Medical Center/ Morgan Stanley Children's Hospital, New York, NY, USA

Anna K. Wright, PhD Neuroscience Institute, Virginia Mason Medical Center, Seattle, WA, USA

Vijay Yanamadala, MD, MBA Department of Neurosurgery, Montefiore Medical Center and Albert Einstein College of Medicine, The Bronx, NY, USA

Center for Surgical Optimization, Leo M. Davidoff Department of Neurosurgery, Montefiore Medical Center, The Bronx, NY, USA

Reza Yassari, MD, MS Department of Neurosurgery, Montefiore Medical Center and Albert Einstein College of Medicine, The Bronx, NY, USA

Macro Trends in Healthcare Delivery

1

Stephen L. Ondra

Healthcare in the United States and around the world is going through a historic transformation. This change is disrupting business models and planning, not only in the way that healthcare is delivered but across a space that intersects with virtually every sector of the economy and has an impact on every individual. Many of the changes taking place may seem chaotic, but if one steps back and looks at several macro trends in healthcare, there is a signal that can be found in the noise that can help us understand where things are moving and how to create a strategy and plan for success.

In this chapter we will explore three broad areas where macro trends are driving change in our healthcare system: cost, consolidation, and new technology. The macro trends in each area will be explored in depth to see how each is impacting the healthcare space; how they relate to each other; how they combine in ways that will change how medicine is practiced and healthcare is delivered; and also how we can achieve the goal of a more accessible, equitable, and affordable healthcare system that is both high in quality and economically sustainable for the nation.

S. L. Ondra (✉)
North Star Healthcare Consulting, LLC, Williston, FL, USA

© Springer Nature Switzerland AG 2020
R. K. Sethi et al. (eds.), *Value-Based Approaches to Spine Care*,
https://doi.org/10.1007/978-3-030-31946-5_1

The Spiraling Cost of Healthcare

Spending on healthcare has reached unsustainable levels in the United States and is hurtling toward a crisis. In 2018, US healthcare expenditures reached $3.7 trillion (T), accounting for 17.8% of our gross domestic product (GDP). This is all the more alarming as the rates continue to increase. The Centers for Medicare and Medicaid Services (CMS) actuaries predict US health spending to reach more than $5.7 T by 2026, eclipsing the 20% of GDP threshold (Fig. 1.1) [1, 2]. CMS also projects that the Medicare Trust Fund will run out of resources to cover expenses by 2026 unless action is taken to avert the current trend in cost.

The short-term and long-term implications for the nation and the federal budget are profound. The US government is now pro-

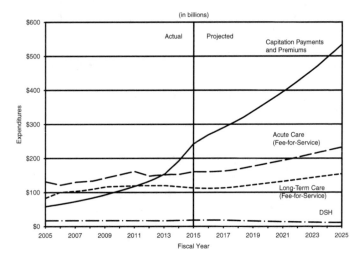

Fig. 1.1 Historical data and projections for Medicaid benefit expenditures for four major categories of services: acute care fee-for-service, long-term care fee-for-service, capitation payments and premiums, and disproportionate share hospital (DSH). The expenditures are in billions of dollars. (Adapted from 2016 Actuarial Report on the Financial Outlook for Medicaid, https://www.cms.gov/Research-Statistics-Data-and-Systems/Research/Actuarial-Studies/Downloads/MedicaidReport2016.pdf)

viding 40% of the overall healthcare coverage and is responsible for 50% of the total healthcare spend. By 2026, these numbers are expected to increase to 48% of all coverage and 60% of the overall health spending in the United States [3].

Two of the most significant reasons for the current fiscal problems are high cost of individual services and intensity of services delivered at the first healthcare encounter. The latter is in large part due to a misalignment of incentives. In the volume-driven fee-for-service (FFS) reimbursement model that dominates healthcare in the United States, the incentive is to get the best outcome possible, but there is little reward for efficient use of resources to achieve that goal. In fact, resource efficiency can be counter to the business interests of those delivering care. In general, the greater the volume of services delivered to the patient, the greater the revenue generation.

While the incentives for delivering quality healthcare include professional integrity, standards of care, peer review, and the medical legal system, the reimbursement incentives often run counter to efficiency. In the volume-driven FFS environment the business and care models are aligned to delivering outcomes in a way that optimizes the throughput of patient services and not necessarily in the most efficient use of resources or the lowest cost of care approach to get to an outcome. This should be no surprise, as behavior is generally guided by the incentives that are provided to individuals and organizations.

This situation is exacerbated by the fact that normal forces that balance a capitalist market economy are largely absent in the healthcare industry. Unlike other market sectors, neither the provider of the services (doctors and hospitals) nor the receiver of those services (patients) are exposed to the actual costs due to the shielding of third-party payment and payment information.

Additionally, neither the provider nor the receiver of services has any direct responsibility for or consequence related to the overall cost of healthcare for the total population. In fact, healthcare culture has long been guided by a single-minded commitment and focus to their responsibility to each individual and not to the cost of care or the impact on the overall cost to society. Population health and global budgets have traditionally had

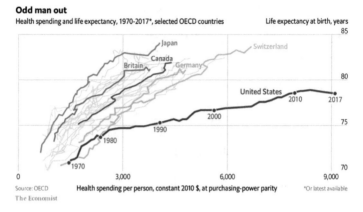

Odd man out

Health spending and life expectancy, 1970-2017*, selected OECD countries

Fig. 1.2 Life expectancy vs. health expenditure over time (1970–2014). (From Max Roser, ourworldindata.org, https://ourworldindata.org/life-expectancy)

secondary concerns, if they were considered at all. This is an idealistic approach, but in the long run, economically unrealistic and ultimately will be dangerous to patients.

The combination of these incentives inherent to the FFS model and the disconnect between normal capitalist cost stabilizing forces have created high in quality but low in value healthcare system in the United States (Fig. 1.2).

The impending economic crisis in healthcare that is coming in the next 5–7 years is largely due to this low-value reality of our healthcare system. Of course, almost everyone looks for where the blame for this situation should lie and who is to blame. While fingers are generally pointed at others as the culprit, the hard truth is that there really is no villain in this story. Every actor from across the healthcare space is simply acting rationally from their point of view, influenced by individual incentives. In fact, not doing that would be a violation of their fiduciary duty to their businesses, employees, or shareholders. In addition to making rational decisions from a business point of view, stakeholders from across the healthcare spectrum are also generally doing what they believe is right for the patient as well as their own business and rational self-interest. As a result, everyone bearing some responsibility for the problem will be impacted by the future solutions.

In addition to understanding the impact of the rational self-interests of all involved, the ongoing presence of some type of third-party payment in healthcare and the resulting disconnect from the normal controls of the capitalist economic model will continue. This is because the idea of solving the problem by moving to a more capitalistic system, where the receiver of services is directly responsible for the costs, is socially unacceptable and economically unrealistic. For most Americans, even the cost of a moderate illness would not be affordable without insurance. In fact, healthcare costs continue to be the leading cause of bankruptcy among those who do not have insurance and for a large percentage of those who do.

As a result, the vast majority of the nation (>80%) believe that health insurance coverage is essential and should be a basic right, with almost two out of three (60%) believing that government should provide coverage, if needed [4, 5]. With that in mind, the continuation of healthcare reimbursement by some third party will continue.

Given this ongoing disconnect between normal balancing economic forces, the most realistic way to solve the unsustainable spiral of healthcare cost is to find new ways of aligning providers and patient incentives, with the ultimate goal of providing high-quality care outcomes, delivered in the most efficient way possible. This is the definition of high-value care as defined by Michael Porter (quality/cost = value) [6].

While there is a need to align economic incentives to value, in order to keep healthcare costs at a sustainable level, there are two important caveats to how this value equation is implemented in order to ensure that patient care is not compromised in a simple race to the bottom on cost. First, the numerator can never be allowed to get smaller, and second, the absolute number of the value equation must get larger or stay the same.

With the value equation as a guiding principle, both public and private payers are demonstrating commitment to finding ways of moving away from the volume-driven FFS reimbursement and toward some form of value-based reimbursement (VBR) that will align incentives to the desired goal of high-quality care delivered as cost efficiently as possible. In the following sections, we will look at some of the initial approaches to VBR, along with their results. In addition, we will discuss how they are continuing to be pushed forward and accelerated by both the payers and purchasers of healthcare.

Models of Value-Based Reimbursement

While the concept of VBR is not new, the initial catalyst to shift from FFS to VBR came from the government and its considerable power as a market maker through CMS. In 2010, the Affordable Care Act (ACA) became the law of the land, and as a part of that law, the Center for Medicare and Medicaid Innovation (CMMI) was formed. The purpose of CMMI was to promote and advance the development, implementation, and propagation of alternative payment models that are aligned to value.

CMMI advanced several VBR models to assess which would be most effective and in what setting. The primary models were the Accountable Care Organization (ACO), Bundled Payments for Care Improvement (BPCI) , and the Patient-Centered Medical Home (PCMH). We will look at each of these, their early results, and what can be expected as VBR continues to mature and expand.

Accountable Care Organization (ACO)

In recent years, ACO has been the most widely used model of VBR. CMS definition of an ACO is "an organization of health care practitioners that agrees to be accountable for the quality, cost, and overall care of Medicare beneficiaries who are enrolled in the traditional fee-for-service program who are assigned to it" [7].

In the ACO model, providers can take upside or upside and downside risk for their population. In upside only risk, care bonus payments are given to providers that meet agreed-upon performance metrics. Failure does not incur a penalty beyond a possible potential upfront reimbursement hold back. Alternatively, ACOs that have downside risk, also referred to as "two-sided risk," provide greater possible reimbursement increases from meeting performance metrics but also have the risk of penalties and paybacks for failure to achieve performance goals. Lastly, there are some ACO models that have a combination of upside and downside risks.

There are many complexities and challenges to implementing an ACO. Providers and payers must agree on metrics, patient inclusion, and provider assignment. Performance measurement can be difficult to calculate, as is the calculation of how the gain from shared savings and assignment of responsibility between providers are adjudicated.

Perhaps the greatest challenge to the success of the ACO model in delivering the optimal potential in value is the lack of patient engagement. Unlike an HMO, patients are usually unaware that they have been assigned to a provider ACO patient panel and bear no responsibility related to it. As a result, up to half of the care received by a population that is assigned to an ACO occurs outside of the contract. This is a major limitation on the provider's ability to control and optimize coordination of care and, with that, the willingness to accept downside risk has been limited.

Additionally, since ACOs are primarily directed at population health and are by nature very primary care focused. Specialists who provide just over half of all care and drive the majority of healthcare spending often find it difficult to see how they fit into this particular VBR model.

While the above challenges have provided obstacles to ACOs reaching their full potential for value improvement, the greatest obstacle is the percentage of a provider's business that is involved in VBR. To realize the full potential of an ACO, or any VBR model, the provider care model must shift to one that is aligned with care quality and cost efficiency and not FFS volume. If an ACO is a minority aspect of the provider's total book of business and the majority of care remains in FFS, there is little incentive for the provider to invest in reinventing the care model and making the investments needed to align with the VBR initiative. In fact, doing so might even degrade their dominant FFS business margins.

Despite these many obstacles and challenges, ACOs have continued to grow in number and covered lives. At the end of 2018, there are over 1000 ACOs in the country, covering 33 million lives. They have not only returned high-quality care but seem to have turned the corner to provide savings in both Medicare and private-payer-sponsored programs.

While increasingly successful, the savings have been less than anticipated and remain a small fraction of the overall healthcare spend. Typical savings have been in the low single-digit percentages when compared to performance of FFS reimbursement (Table 1.1). When compared with the consistent double-digit savings seen in many HMOs, up to 20% year over year when compared to the broad PPO networks, ACO performance may seem disappointing, but it should be remembered that we are early in experience with ACOs and they will continue to be refined and improved and are more broadly scalable than the HMO model. It is expected that over time, ACOs will not only continue to expand but will come closer to realizing their full potential for value improvement [8].

Table 1.1 CMS assessment of Medicare Shared Saving Programs (MSSP) performance from 2012/2013 through 2017

MSSP cohort (based on start year)	Net savings (loss) to Medicare (after shared savings payments to ACOs)
2012/2013	$205 million
2014	$173 million
2015	$5 million
2016	$34 million
2017	$34 million
Total	$314 million

Data from https://www.cms.gov/Medicare/Medicare-Fee-for-Service-Payment/sharedsavingsprogram/index.html?redirect=/sharedsavingsprogram/

Bundled Payment of Care Improvement (BPCI)

The Bundled Payments of Care Improvement (BPCI) and BPCI Advanced programs focus on linking multiple providers and services to payments for a disease-specific episode of care. These programs have been targeted at specific high-cost diagnostic categories, and while primary care does participate in care bundles, it is a more specialist-oriented model than the ACO programs. While it has the disadvantage of being more limited in broad population impact, it has the advantage of being targeted where it will have the most near-term impact on cost and value improvement. BPCI programs also have the benefit of providing near-term measurable endpoints that are relevant to the business cycle time frames of all stakeholders [9]. This is often in the time frame of 1- to 3-year results.

CMS has pushed forward a number of models in recent years, targeting such conditions as joint replacement and congestive heart failure. These models have many of the same challenges that were discussed when reviewing ACOs, such as agreement on metrics, inclusion and exclusion criteria, patient assignment, and gain sharing between participants and participant organizations. Also, the percentage of practice that is in the bundle must be sufficient enough to reach enough of a critical mass that it makes business sense to not simply participate but to also modify the FFS tuned care model. It is at that point that the incentives to invest in both the infrastructure and cultural change managment will be sufficient to realize the full potential of BPCI models.

Lastly, changes in government policy in 2017 created uncertainty in the future of the program. This resulted in enough uncertainty that annual corporate budgets scaled back BPCI-related provider and payer planning and investments, which delayed progress 2–3 years from what was predicted. CMS has now shifted policy back to expanding BPCI programs. As a result, interest has again increased and BPCI programs are growing in number and scope.

With similar challenges to ACOs, it is no surprise that BPCI performance results have also been mixed for CMS. For lower extremity joint replacement, CMS showed a lowering of expected cost by an average of 4.5%. In the congestive heart failure bundle, costs were decreased by 3.6% [10].

Despite this limited early performance success, the private sector has begun to push for increased utilization of the BPCI programs. Frustrated by traditional payer inability to control and/ or stabilize healthcare costs, increasing numbers of private sector self-insured employers are beginning to carve out BPCI contracts from their private payer administrative service only (ASO) agreements [11]. This, in turn, is putting pressure on traditional health insurers to become more innovative and aggressive on VBR programs in general and BPCI programs in particular.

It is expected that BPCI programs will continue to grow in the number and scope of covered conditions. With additional experience and sophistication and as critical mass in these contracts is reached, along with the expected continuation of cuts in FFS reimbursement, participation in BPCI will not only grow but will increase the value created by these programs.

Patient-Centered Medical Home (PCMH)

The Patient-Centered Medical Home (PCMH) programs are high-touch initiatives with greatest use in narrowly defined populations of high-risk, high-frequency healthcare users. While the narrow focus of these programs makes them easier to administer in many ways, the high cost of operating this care model makes it impractical for all broad populations. Despite this limitation, the reality that 5% of patients accounting for up to 50% of healthcare costs provide an opportunity to identify specific populations and programs that would benefit from such a high touch model and as a result, significantly increase outcome quality and reduce overall cost through readmission avoidance and other impacts. In addition to reducing healthcare costs, employers and patients find benefit in targeting these high-risk populations with high-touch PCMH programs that reduce lost work days and improve employee productivity.

Despite these advantages and some notable successes, the more narrow population and difficulty in running unique programs for targeted populations has resulted in more limited use for this approach to VBR. This combined with the all too frequent overgeneralization of the PCMH model and the predictable associated disappointing results has reduced interest, use, and impact for PCMHs.

Despite this, the PCMH model is well suited for specific populations and may yet prove to be an important part of a portfolio of VBR tools that can be deployed to a population in a targeted way and then combined together to form a composite VBR approach.

Summary of VBR Models

In the end, it should be no surprise that the initial VBR models have had disappointing results. Most new programs of any kind go through a period of refinement and modification as theory meets the reality of implementation. The initial challenges faced by the current VBR models should be seen as an opportunity to learn and improve on these approaches in order to deliver on their full potential and address the need for increased healthcare value.

In addition to VBR program refinement, as mentioned earlier, the "critical mass effect" will be another potential tipping point to realize the potential of VBR to drive overall positive change in our health system. Once provider's contract percentage in VBR reaches between 35% and 50% threshold, the business incentive for investing in infrastructure and the culture change needed to alter the care model in a way that will allow the full benefits of care coordination will be reached.

Lastly, while it would appear simpler to pick one VBR model to drive change, the reality is that healthcare delivery in a large and diverse nation means that a one size fits all model is unrealistic. Variations in provider specialties, practice patterns, dominant practice business environments, and the geographic differences, all impact the care delivery and what might be the best fit for a VBR model.

A more practical approach will be to have a defined set of VBR models and over time identify the characteristics of providers that have the best chance for success in each model. Once that is done, a model that best fits the capabilities and needs for a market can be identified. This would result in the least disruption for the greatest return. Over time, various models can evolve in a way that will allow them to fit together to create a mosaic of value improvement. While this lacks the elegance and optimization of a fully planned system, it has the practicality needed to implement change in a large and complex environment that involves one sixth of our economy and is still deeply engrained in the FFS business and care delivery models.

Other Macroeconomic Trends

While the transition to VBR is usually the primary focus of discussion, there are other drivers of profound change that are impacting the healthcare system and are a part of an ecosystem of change.

Price Controls and Decreases in Reimbursement

There is a general agreement that we must shift from the current volume-driven FFS reimbursement model to one that aligns with stakeholder incentives for higher value; however, many obstacles have meant that change is happening far more slowly than needed.

Payers may have the ability and tools to drive this change, but the simple truth is that private insurers and everyone else in the healthcare sector are still making enough money that there is no rational business reason to go through the cost, effort, and organizational change management needed for a large-scale disruptive transition to their business.

Another reality that has slowed the transition from FFS to VBR is that the return on investment for population health must be in a time frame that is relevant to the insurer or the employer, and that is only as long as the average time that an employee remains with an employer or a beneficiary remains with an insurer. According to the Bureau of Labor Statistics report published in 2018, the average time that an employee stays with a company is 4.6 years. Health plans do not anticipate consumer loyalty for more than 1–2 years. This often creates a mismatch between good public policy, which looks at lifetime cycles, and the private sector coverage groups that need to see a return on population health investments within 1–5 years.

This, along with the considerable implementation challenges, has resulted in the slower than expected transition from FFS to VBR, renewing interest in price cuts and controls for reimbursement in both public and private sector payers/purchasers [12]. The expected round of price cuts will squeeze already thin margins even further for providers, further stressing an already stressed system for the providers and vendors of care delivery products.

The result of the expected further cuts in FFS reimbursement will change the calculation on the difficulty and merits of investing in changing reimbursement models and will further align the interests that are accelerating change.

Consolidation

To gain negotiating power with payers, as well as business efficiencies, providers have gone through a dramatic increase in mergers and vertical integration (Fig. 1.3), including physicians joining mega-groups, hospital mergers and acquisitions, and hospital-provider mergers. This is a rational action on behalf of providers and provider organizations to address shrinking margins that have resulted from contracted cuts in payer reimbursement.

While this has been good for providers, this vertical integration has consistently resulted in higher costs for payers, consumers, and the nation as a whole [13, 14]. Provider mergers and vertical integration has resulted in a reaction from the payer and employer/purchaser communities. We are now seeing vertical integration in the payers and pharma sectors, with such mergers as CVS and Aetna. Also, payers have begun to acquire provider groups in a

Hospital Mergers on the Rise

Health care providers may seek to blunt
competition by consolidating. Over the past
decade, the annual number of hospital mergers
in the U.S. has doubled.

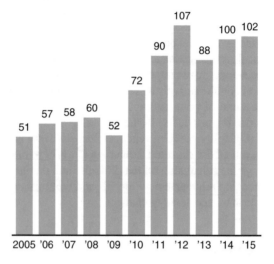

Fig. 1.3 Hospital mergers have doubled in the past decade and are continuing despite regulatory concerns and pressure. (From American Hospital Association and Irving Levin Associates. Reprinted with permission from "Health Care Needs Real Competition" by Leemore S. Dafny and Thomas H. Lee. Harvard Business Review, December 2016. Copyright 2016 by Harvard Business Publishing; all rights reserved)

new kind of vertical integration, where incentive alignment to value improvement can be directly managed. Other realignments are expected as nontraditional entities begin to enter the chaotic healthcare sector. The entrance of Amazon and others will be potentially a powerful disruptor that can create new paradigms of care and drive innovation in the traditional healthcare sector incumbents. It is unclear where these realignments, mergers, and joint ventures will lead, but a creative disruption of the traditional stakeholder business models and relationships will continue, providing risk and opportunity.

New Technology

Changes in technology will also be transformative to the healthcare sector in ways that are difficult to predict; however, they have consistently been the cause of fundamental transformation in how care is practiced and delivered. Until now, healthcare has been unique among business sectors in that technology has added rather than reduced cost. This is due to many factors, but again the malalignment of incentives is a major contributor. This malalignment results in business incentives that bring products to market that will not only improve care but are oriented to drive volume-related return on investment, rather than cost reduction and efficiency. A shift to VBR will finally create an incentive to get a return for products that improve care and efficiency of care delivery. The following are a few of the technology sectors where the transition to VBR will provide a more fertile business environment.

Telehealth

Telehealth is already fast becoming a transformative trend in medical practice and care delivery. For a significant subset of care, telehealth has the ability to extend the reach of both primary and specialty care and deliver it to patients in a more convenient and efficient way for both doctor and patient. Until now, the major impediment was not the technology infrastructure, though that continues to rapidly evolve. Rather, the unclear volumes and impact on cost has resulted in a hesitance for payers to add a new channel of FFS reimbursement. The emergence of VBR will create an aligned interest to use this technology to improve care value. Additionally, there are legislative and medical licensing moves that can be made to address some of the regulatory hurdles and promote the development of telehealth [15].

Smart Pharmaceuticals and Devices

New devices and pharmaceuticals are now available that can stream data on use, compliance, performance, location, and a variety of physiologic parameters. This data can be used to understand if patients are taking prescriptions and if their medication is having the desired effect. It can also give insight into the performance of implanted medical devices to provide added insight. Such information can aid in a better understanding of who will benefit the most from various treatment options and will be needed for providers engaged in VBR models to optimize care in a way that will allow them to improve the treatment efficiency needed to succeed in shared risk arrangements.

In addition to traditional VBR models with providers, streaming data can provide the information that would be needed for pharmaceutical and device makers to engage in value-based contracts.

The rapid increase in the cost of pharmaceuticals has driven a keen interest in the concept of linking the sale of pharmaceuticals to the associated outcome. This would incentivize both the pharmaceutical industry and prescriber to target the highest-value treatment to a patient, rather than just incentivizing higher volumes of an appropriate treatment that may or may not be the highest-value alternative.

Aligning incentives to value in the pharmaceutical industry makes sense; however, the difficulty of implementing value-based pharmaceutical contracts, combined with the fact that the discounts currently available have kept the revenue margins high enough for payer, pharmacy benefit manager (PBM), and the pharmaceutical industry, means that the compelling business reason to go through the difficult and costly process of shifting to pharma VBR does not yet exist. Until those margins are changed through government or private sector action, it is unlikely that VBR in the pharmaceutical sector will get traction beyond policy discussion.

With providers largely a pass-through due to third-party pharma payments and in some cases a beneficiary from high prices in areas such as oncology, it is the patient and purchaser/ employer which are the two groups most negatively impacted by the high cost of pharmaceuticals and benefit the least from the web of discounts and contract benefits that the payers, PBMs, and pharma companies engage in. Ultimately, it will be pressure from this sector and government payers that will drive VBR into the pharma sector.

A shift to VBR in the pharmaceutical will create a need for information beyond simply having prescriptions written and refilled. There will be a need to ensure that medication is taken, taken correctly and to obtain ever more personalized information on the profile of which medication is most effective in which patient by the acquisition of real-world performance of pharmaceuticals. That will make smart pills increasingly viable from a business development standpoint.

Similar to the pharmaceuticals, medical devices will likely begin to see pressure to provide guarantees on outcomes and performance that will lead to the possibility of engagement in VBR programs with payers and/or providers as a way to share revenue as well as risk. Again, to be successful in such a model will require more real-time/real-world information on patient status and device performance to identify which patient is most likely to optimally benefit from a specific device and procedure. As in pharmaceuticals, such a business model provides the incentives and return on investment for smart devices.

Closing the loop on alignment of incentives, it should be remembered that the provider who is engaged in a VBR contract will also be powerfully incented to know that their patient is correctly and reliably taking the medication they have been prescribed and/or they have made the best possible personalized choice of medication, procedural intervention, and the devices used in that intervention for that specific patient.

Genetics

The field of genetics and personalized medicine is not an economic trend but is a macro scientific trend that will continue to have a profound impact on how medicine is practiced and healthcare is delivered and how those involved in other sectors of this space operate. The ability to quickly and easily get genetic information on patients at relatively low cost continues to expand. This is opening new possibilities for truly personalized understanding of disease and treatment on an individual, rather than at a population level.

As discussed above, the shift to VBR will heighten the need to specifically target optimal therapies to individual needs. Until now, patients have been lumped together as an entire population or only crudely been divided by age, gender, or other healthcare and population characteristics. While this helps target therapy to some degree, it requires large populations to wash out variable risk and make VBR work. By obtaining data that can allow personalized targeted therapy to an individual, the specific highest-value treatment for each patient can be more easily identified and utilized. This will make VBR easier and more successful in general and also viable in smaller populations.

The ease of genetic testing to target therapies, such as pharmaceuticals, is an example of how genetics and personalized medicine can be an enabler of VBR. For example, statins have been a powerful tool in combating cholesterol and its impact on heart disease. There are many options; and which to prescribe to a patient is largely left to physician preference, impacted by their general experience with the population and other factors. As successful as this has been in the population, it would be even more effective if the statin to be prescribed is matched to that individual's genetic profile in order to ensure that it is the specific drug that will be most effective. Such information will provide doctor and patient with important personalized information, dramatically improve patient health, minimize needless risk, and help VBR models be successful.

The above is just one example, but the understanding of genetics and its impact on disease and treatment is a macro trend in medicine that will have a major impact on disease, treatment, and the economics of healthcare.

Wearable Devices

The last technology trend will be in wearable devices, smart implants, and smart pharmaceuticals that can continuously stream physiologic data from patients. Such data can then be fed to artificial intelligence (AI) engines that can provide real-time, personalized, and actionable information to care providers. This can be used to aid providers in identifying clinical changes, some of which patients may not yet be aware of, and act proactively before illness becomes profound or even present.

Such information can help the care team work with patients in a way that avoids or shortens hospitalization, quickly identify the impact or lack of impact of treatment, and improve the health and lives of patients. Improving health and optimizing treatment will also aid providers in succeeding in the various emerging VBR models. Lastly, such information can inform and empower patients to improve their own health, healthcare, and work with their care team in new and more collaborative ways.

Initially, this will be most practical for populations in which wearable or implanted monitoring devices can be used for those most profoundly impacted by highly morbid chronic diseases. For example 5% of the population that account for 50% of all healthcare spending. Wearable or implanted devices can be used initially in patients who have the most morbid chronic conditions and would most benefit from continuous monitoring in terms of improved outcome and a lower all cost of care. As the price of wearable devices and monitoring goes down in the near future, and AI algorithms become ever smarter and more capable of seamlessly fitting into the care teams workflow, the ability of such insight to move into common use will be possible.

Accessing real-time streamed physiological data and converting the data into usable information will be another of the many emerging technologies that will transform healthcare treatment and its payment models.

Big Data and Artificial Intelligence

Almost all of the macro trends in healthcare economics and the mega trends in technology are dependent on the mountains of "big data" that are being generated and can be used by machine learning-driven artificial intelligence (AI). The use of AI and AI engines to generate information is the most profound potential disruptor to the status quo in healthcare and society at large. It is also a powerful enabler of change.

AI will provide real-time insights that can enable the shift to VBR in a more practical, accurate, and successful way. It will also change the nature of medical practice and how patients interact with their care teams.

While "big data" and AI will profoundly impact and help to transform the entire healthcare space, from payment to practice, those changes will in turn impact on the healthcare technology infrastructure development. One example is the current and often frustrating electronic health records (EHRs) that are commonly in use today.

Like the rest of healthcare, the current generation of EHRs is tuned to support the current FFS revenue cycle management financial model. The information generated is much more helpful to managing the business of healthcare than the delivery of it. As a result, physicians and other providers of care often feel that they are spending too much time as data entry technicians for the EHR than they are actually helped by it in the care of patients. A shift to VBR will force the current EHRs to become more oriented and optimized for care delivery efficiency. When this occurs, there will be a market demand shift that will push legacy EHR providers to transform their products. Such a transition will open opportunities for new entrants that are purpose built to provide care teams with the type of interface and information that they will need to succeed in improving care and care value.

Conclusion: Finding Signal in the Noise

While all of the change in public policy, business, and technology makes the healthcare system seem chaotic, some consistent signals are emerging. It is not any one of these signals that will determine the overall change that is coming to the massive healthcare sector. Rather, it will be a combination of the various macroeconomic forces that are poised to dramatically change the business and care models for every sector of the healthcare space and how they relate to each other.

In the near term, the slow pace of transition to VBR has resulted in a continuation of the unsustainable spiral of healthcare costs. As a result, another round of cuts in reimbursement prices is likely. This in turn will reduce margins and be an additional catalyst to speed the transition to VBR.

The steady transition away from FFS and toward VBR models will hit a tipping point, at which time the transition will become rapid. This will not be in a single one size fits all but rather a defined portfolio of options that payers and providers can engage in ways that fit their capabilities and needs.

Similarly, various options used in a market will be in a combination that is best suited to the needs and patterns that are present in each regional market. This portfolio of VBR options will continue to evolve as experience and technology begin to provide the knowledge and tools for refinement and the assembly of a mosaic of approaches to improve health outcomes and lower cost.

The shift in the fundamental business model underlying the massive healthcare space will take time, but as the shift from FFS to VBR occurs, technology that is being refined today will aid in enabling and catalyzing that shift and will in turn be shaped by it.

The profound change that is in relative slow motion now but will continue to gain momentum. It will be wise to begin to gain experience in the systems and processes that will be needed for success in VBR but are usable in current business operations. The smart choice will be in extensible systems and processes that will minimize the need for wholesale restructuring when the transition to VBR becomes a major or the dominant model.

The growing role of government in the coverage and payment of healthcare, combined with the growing deficit in the federal budget, will mean that there is likely to be another major government action if and when a crisis is reached. That time is likely in the next 5–10 years, and a good bet is that will be when the Medicare Trust Fund is at risk of running out of funds to cover costs. That is now projected for 2026, the same year that healthcare costs are likely to approach $6 T. What action will be politically possible is unclear, but it is notable that both the Obama and Trump Administrations have continued to pursue VBR as one of the best solution to controlling costs and covering high-quality care. That makes it likely that VBR will be a goal of any legislation, regardless of the political landscape.

Transitioning from the current business model to one that aligns incentives across the stakeholders in the healthcare space to deliver higher value will likely result in disruption of business and care models that will create winners and losers in a sector that was previously almost only had winners. The winners are likely to be those that are adaptable and not philosophically rigid. The winners are most likely to be those who choose to plan, make the investments in tools and culture in a way that will allow them to gain the experience that will lay a groundwork for operating today but also be adaptable to the likely needs of the future.

References

1. 2016 Actuarial report on the financial outlook for Medicaid. 2016.
2. Meyer H. Healthcare spending will hit 19.4% of GDP in the next decade, CMS projects. Modern Healthcare. 2019 February 20.
3. Conover C. The Federal share of American health spending is now approaching 50%. Forbes.
4. Bialik K. More Americans say government should ensure health care coverage. Universal Health Care. 2018:94.
5. Jajich-Toth C, Roper BW. Americans' views on health care: a study in contradictions. Health Aff. 1990;9(4):149–57.
6. Porter ME. What is value in health care? N Engl J Med. 2010;363(26):2477–81.
7. Accountable Care Organizations (ACO) [updated 03/08/2019]. Available from: https://www.cms.gov/Medicare/Medicare-Fee-for-Service-Payment/ACO/.
8. Pathways to success: a new start for Medicare's Accountable Care Organization. Health affairs blog. August 9, 2018.
9. Bundled Payments for Care Improvement (BPCI) Initiative: general information [updated 4/17/2019. Available from: https://innovation.cms.gov/initiatives/bundled-payments/.
10. Haefner M. CMS releases annual report on bundled payment performance: 5 things to know. Becker's Hospital CFO Report. 2017.
11. Japsen B. Employers accelerate move to value-based care in 2018. Forbes. 2017.
12. Meyer H. Why does the U.S. spend so much more on healthcare? It's the prices. Modern Healthcare. 2018.
13. Gooch K. Hospital mergers often raise prices, analysis finds. Becker's Hospital CFO Report. 2018.
14. LaPointe J. Do Hospital Mergers, acquisitions increase prices, reps ask MedPAC revcycle intelligence 2018. Available from: https://revcycleintelligence.com/news/do-hospital-mergers-acquisitions-increase-prices-reps-ask-medpac.
15. Sweeney E. House Committee passes bill to build telehealth coverage into medicare advantage plans. Fierce Healthcare [Internet]. 2017. Available from: https://www.fiercehealthcare.com/regulatory/house-committee-unanimously-passes-bill-to-make-telehealth-part-basic-coverage-medicare.

Evaluating Policy Effects in the Treatment of Lumbar Fusion

2

Brook I. Martin, Sohail K. Mirza, and Daniel J. Finch

Background

Facing increasing questions concerning the value of lumbar spinal fusion for certain indications, payers have frequently targeted the procedure for coverage and reimbursement reform, a practice that has modified utilization and outcomes [1]. Consequently, population-based studies using state and national data strive to quantify and document the effects that these policies can have on healthcare resource utilization and safety. Despite their limitations, the use of state and national databases, such as the Agency for Healthcare Research and Quality's National Inpatient Sample (NIS) and the State Inpatient Database (SID), are perhaps the only

B. I. Martin (✉)
Department of Orthopaedic, University of Utah,
Salt Lake City, UT, USA
e-mail: u6011700@utah.edu

S. K. Mirza
Department of Orthopaedic, Dartmouth-Hitchcock Medical Center,
Lebanon, NH, USA

D. J. Finch
Department of Orthopaedic, University of Utah,
Salt Lake City, UT, USA

Tufts University, Boston, MA, USA

© Springer Nature Switzerland AG 2020
R. K. Sethi et al. (eds.), *Value-Based Approaches to Spine Care*,
https://doi.org/10.1007/978-3-030-31946-5_2

practical means for understanding the effect of policy modifications at population level. Analysis of hospital administrative data, which typically include diagnosis and procedure codes, to measure specific outcomes requires linking successive spine-related claims for a target patient population over time to describe healthcare utilization, treatment pathway, and episode of care costs. Algorithms based on Current Procedural Terminology (CPT) and International Classification of Disease (versions 9 and 10) diagnosis and procedure codes have been validated to for characterizing spine-related medical encounters into clinically meaningful diagnoses and for describing manual, percutaneous, imaging, and surgical procedures, as well as vertebral regions, and operative features [2–5]. These algorithms have been used to describe trends in operative and nonoperative procedures, resource utilization, surgical invasiveness, safety indicators, and the effects of adopting evidence-based practice policies. Several case studies have emerged in recent years that exemplify this approach, and studies validating and improving the implementation of claims-based research have advanced these efforts.

Rates and Trends of Lumbar Fusion

Indications for spinal fusion are varied and unevenly applied. The procedure is established for spinal deformity, fracture, and instability. However, the evidence of effectiveness is more controversial for other indications, including disc herniation and degeneration, nonspecific back pain, and spinal stenosis without instability. While the prevalence of spinal pathologies is not known, the rates of lumbar fusion continue to rise [6]. The volume of elective lumbar fusion increased 62.3% (from 122,679 cases to 199,140 cases) between 2004 and 2015, exceeding procedure growth explained solely by population increase. The rise in volume is especially notable in the patients aged 65 or older, demonstrating the increasing willingness of surgeons to operate on older adults (Fig. 2.1). The largest increases in surgical volumes were for indications of spondylolisthesis (spinal instability) and scoliosis (a spinal deformity), but the more controversial indica-

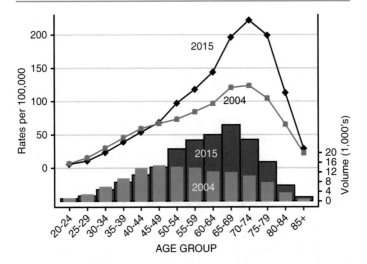

Fig. 2.1 Age-specific trends in population rates (per 100,000 adults, left axis) and volume (1000's of procedures, right axis) of elective inpatient lumbar fusion operations for degenerative diagnoses in the United States, 2004 and 2015. Estimates based on survey-weighted Poisson regression including covariates for year, age, and sex. (From Martin et al. [6], with permission). *Source*: Nationwide Inpatient Sample (NIS) 2004–2015

tions of disc degeneration, herniation, and stenosis still combined to account for a significant number of elective lumbar fusions. As the utility of fusion for degeneration, herniation, and stenosis are increasingly questioned and payers are less inclined to pay for these operations, the proportion of fusion procedures performed for these indications has decreased from 58% of total fusions in 2004 to 42% in 2015. Along with the increase in spinal fusion volume, the aggregate national hospital costs of inpatient spinal fusions have increased from $8.6 billion in 2004 to $24 billion in 2015, including a 70% increase in per-case cost from roughly $30,000 to $52,000. Fusions involving disc herniation, disc degeneration, and spinal stenosis amounted to over $10 billion in 2015, about 40% of total elective lumbar spinal fusion costs. With imprecise indications, wide-ranging pathologies, and growing costs, it is little wonder that spinal fusion procedures are often targeted for payment reform.

Washington State Worker Compensation System

In 2006, Washington State's worker compensation (WC) program, managed through the Department of Labor and Industry, revised its policies to place restrictions on lumbar fusion for unilateral disc herniation, multiple vertebral levels, and complex circumferential approaches. The policy included a prospective utilization review for all fusions, imaging confirmation of spinal instability, and limited fusion procedures to a single disc level. During the same period, California's workers' compensation system only relied on a binding second opinion authorization and provided additional payments for stabilizing instrumentation in adjacent vertebrae and bone-growth enhancement. Population-level cross-sectional comparison of utilization, costs, and 3-month safety, using the Agency for Healthcare Research and Quality's (AHRQ) State Inpatient Database (SID), explored the effects of these different state-specific coverage policies [7]. Interestingly, the overall rate of lumbar fusion operations among WC patients was 47% higher in California than in Washington State. In addition, California WC patients were significantly more likely than those in Washington to undergo fusion for nonspecific back pain (28% versus 21%) or disc herniation (37% versus 21%), as opposed to more widely accepted indications, including spinal stenosis (6% versus 15%), and spondylolisthesis (25% versus 41%). Strikingly, patients in California had a significantly higher adjusted risk for undergoing a reoperation (relative risk [RR] 2.28; 95%; Fig. 2.2). Differences in demographic or clinical characteristics do not explain the difference in complications. Instead, they are likely attributed to the refined indications and the reduced use of combined approaches, multilevel fusions, stabilizing instrumentation, and bone morphogenetic protein in Washington State. These findings suggest that less restrictive coverage policies are associated with more aggressive practice styles, leading to greater rates of reoperation, readmission, and complications.

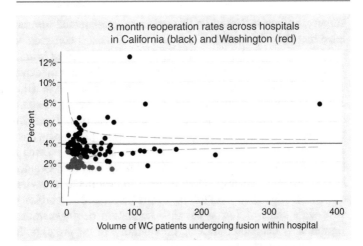

Fig. 2.2   Rates of repeat lumbar surgery within 3 months among hospitals performing lumbar fusion operations among worker compensation patients, State Inpatient Database 2008–2009 combined. Each point represents a single hospital from California (black) or Washington (red). The horizontal solid line represents the overall mean for all hospitals. (From Martin et al. [7]; with permission). *Source:* State Inpatient Database, 2008–2009. Adjusted for age, sex, comorbidity, and diagnosis. Horizontal black line represents overall mean. Dashed funnel plots represent 95% CI control limits

Blue Cross Blue Shield of North Carolina Policy

In addition to state-level programs, other payers in healthcare, including large commercial insurers, have attempted to use reimbursement to guide clinical practice in spinal fusion. There is evidence that fusion surgery is effective for treating unstable spondylolisthesis, fracture, or scoliosis. However, there is limited evidence that fusion provides any advantage over nonoperative care in treating degenerative disc disease or that adding fusion to decompression procedures improves outcomes for patients with disc herniation or spinal stenosis. Indeed, unnecessary fusion exposes patients to the risk of complication, repeat surgery, and costs. Based on this evidence, commercial insurers have increasingly sought to limit the use of what it considers to be the inappropriate use of lumbar fusion by restricting insurer payments for indications where there is relatively weak evidence of clinical effectiveness. In January of 2011, Blue Cross Blue Shield of North Carolina refused to provide coverage of lumbar fusion where the sole indication was disc herniation, degenerative disc, or stenosis without spondylolisthesis [1]. Time-series data from North Carolina's State Inpatient Database showed a highly specific reduction in the use of fusion for these targeted indications and a corresponding increase in decompression without fusion (Fig. 2.3). Controlling for age, sex, and comorbidity, state-wide rates of fusion for disc herniation or degeneration significantly declined following the initiation of the program. In North Carolina, lumbar fusion for these two indications increased by an average of 11 cases per year before the implementation of the new Blue Cross Blue Shield policy and decreased by 71

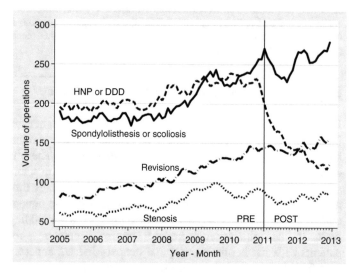

Fig. 2.3 Monthly trend in volume of lumbar fusion surgery in North Carolina by surgical indication, before and after commercial coverage policy change. (From Martin et al. [1]; with permission)

cases per year after the policy was enacted ($p < 0.001$). There was no evidence of a corresponding rise in the rate of fusions for spondylolisthesis, scoliosis, or spinal stenosis, suggesting that patients were not reassigned to covered indications. The decrease in lumbar fusion for disc herniation or degenerative disc disease, without a corresponding increase for other indications, suggests that this policy had its intended effect of reserving fusion operations for indications that have the best support of clinical evidence of effectiveness.

Early Effects of Medicare's Bundled Payment Program for Lumbar Fusion

Lumbar fusion among Medicare beneficiaries is traditionally reimbursed as a fee-for-service payment, which lacks incentives to reward quality, coordination, or effectiveness of care provided. Medicare is experimenting with modifying incentives through bundled payments, which are an alternative reimbursement approach that has gained traction through the Center for Medicare and Medicaid Innovation's (CMMI) Bundled Payment for Care Improvement (BPCI) program. This program establishes a predetermined target payment for all services related to a fusion operation over a defined time period, typically a 90-day "episode-of-care," and is another example of payer reform aimed at shaping clinical care. Hospitals that provide care at costs below the predetermined amount may share in any savings achieved, while those that provide services at costs above the predetermined payment will incur financial loss. An early retrospective analysis of 2012–2013 Medicare claims linked to public reports of hospital participation in CMMI's BPCI program provides some evidence of the preliminary effects of the program. Even after controlling for demographics and comorbidity, reductions in Medicare 90-day episode-of-care costs from 2012 to 2013 were significant among hospitals that did not participate in the BPCI program for lumbar fusion, but were unchanged for participant hospitals (Fig. 2.4). There was a 1.8% ($368) reduction in the 90-day episode-of-care payment for lumbar fusion among non-BPCI hospi-

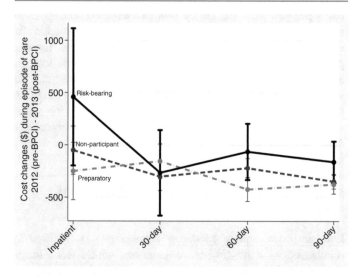

Fig. 2.4 Changes in 90-day episode of care payments from 2012 (pre-BPCI) to 2013 (post-BPCI) based on hospital voluntary participation in the Center for Medicare and Medicaid Innovation's (CMMI) Bundled Payment for Care Improvement (BPCI) program for lumbar fusion. (From Martin et al. [8], with permission)

tals, from $20,389 in 2012 to $20,021 in 2013. Of concern, from 2012 to 2013, all-cause readmission and repeat spine surgery rates significantly worsened among BPCI participant hospitals compared to readmission and reoperation among nonparticipants. The concerning early findings that BPCI participant hospitals failed to achieve a decrease in the mean episode payment during the year following program initiation of the program, combined with the alarming increase in readmissions, provide early evidence that BPCI's program for lumbar fusion might be ineffective at reducing costs and improving the quality of care received.

Epidemiology of Bone Morphogenetic Protein in Lumbar Fusion

Payers are not the only groups that influence clinical practice in spinal fusion. The Agency for Healthcare Research and Quality's (AHRQ) National Inpatient Sample (NIS) is useful to investigate how providers alter clinical practice in response to evolving evidence of safety and effectiveness. For example, the use of recombinant human bone morphogenetic protein-2 (BMP) as an adjunct to spinal fusion surgery proliferated following its Food and Drug Administration (FDA) approval in 2002. Although approved as an adjunct for single-level anterior lumbar fusion, its off-label use proliferated to other procedures, including posterior, interbody, and cervical fusions. A monthly time-series regression analysis documents the initial rapid increase in the proportion of spinal fusion procedures involving BMP, followed by its statistically significant decrease following a 2008 FDA public health notification raising safety concerns and accompanying revelations of finan-

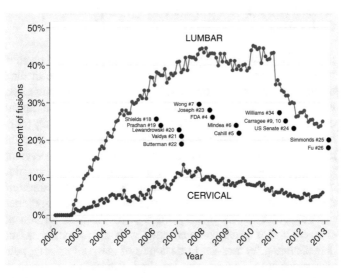

Fig. 2.5 US trends in the percent of lumbar and cervical fusion operations involving bone morphogenetic proteins in relationship to published safety reports. (From Martin et al. [9], with permission)

cial conflicts of interests among surgeons involved in the FDA-approved trials (Fig. 2.5) [9]. These revelations brought to light by that US Senate Finance Committee investigation that concluded that "Medtronic was involved in drafting, editing, and shaping the content of medical journal articles authored by its physician consultants who received significant amounts of money through royalties and consulting fees from Medtronic." A subsequent independent reanalysis of the FDA data concluded that BMP had no clinical advantage over iliac crest bone graft and that its risks were understated in published reports. An *Annals of Internal Medicine* editorial stated that "Early journal publications misrepresented the effectiveness and harms through selective reporting, duplicate publication, and underreporting." This infamous episode in spinal fusion history underscored the importance of using national-level data to observe and analyze the epidemiology and trends in orthopedic procedures in response to changing research findings, government investigations, and policy modifications.

Where Are Spine Policies Going: Emphasizing Outcomes

Historically, quality assurance in medicine has been based on clinical credentialing, such as through the Joint Commission, medical board specialty and subspecialty, licensure, continuing education, and affiliation through professional societies. Under the current environment of healthcare reform, this paradigm is rapidly shifting. Increasingly, quality assurance requires an understanding the end results of treatment. Quality includes measuring the structure, process, and outcomes in the system of care, comparing hospital and surgeon performance, and emphasizing timely, real-world, and comprehensive analysis centered on meaningful patient-reported outcomes. The quality paradigm recognizes the need for clinical efficacy studies to be complemented with translational research demonstrating the real-world outcomes of new and existing policies, procedures, devices, and practices. Clinical management of spine disease has not kept pace with these changing expectations. For example, even as the focus shifts to understanding factors that lead to improved patient outcomes, standardized, validated, and well-accepted measures of patient-reported outcomes remain elusive to researchers, policymakers, and surgeons in the spine field. Policymakers and field leaders are challenged with improving the value of care through better outcomes and reduced costs without being able to quantify or assess long-term patient outcomes easily. Patient-reported outcomes must be longitudinally collected, analyzed, and reported to help understand the value of certain types of medical care, especially invasive and expensive treatments like spine surgery. Our changing health ecosystem emphasizes evidence-based medicine based on high-value care, and measuring and analyzing the end goal of medicine (improved patient outcomes) at the population level is a crucial component of these efforts.

Measuring Quality in Back Pain: Medicare's Hospital Compare and the OP-8 Measure

Medicare's Hospital Compare program [10] provides an example of how the quality of care is measured and shared in spine care. The Hospital Compare website ranks hospitals across the country on numerous quality measures, enabling the public to view data on utilization, complications, mortality, and costs, relative to state and national averages. One of the goals of this project is to encourage hospitals to improve the quality and reduce the costs care, offering an opportunity for hospitals and their affiliated providers to attract patients based on quality and safety measures instead of traditional referral networks.

The use of advanced imaging like MRIs and CTs is one of the fastest growing services reimbursed by Medicare and an aspect of spine care that has proliferated since 2000. Hospital Compare data includes publicly available information about outpatient MRI use without antecedent conservative care. This measure, the Outpatient Imaging Efficiency Measure 8 ("OP-8") is a proxy measure for overutilization of MRIs for low back pain. In the context of spinal care, an MRI for low back pain can return false-positive and anomalous findings that may lead to spine surgery. Interestingly, research found that the implementation and public reporting of this measure did not result in decreased MR imaging rates for low back pain without prior conservative therapy, even under financial pressures to do so [11].

The OP-8 measure helps represent both the possibilities and complexities of comparing hospital-level utilization measures in spine care based on claims data. Continued modifications of the OP-8 measure Medicare were necessary after flaws in the methodology of compiling the measure were noted. For example, the measure does not seem to fully account for imaging indications based on age, clinical context, or personal characteristics of each patient [12]. While overutilization of costly imaging is a valid concern for both providers and payers, valid and clinically useful measures that compare hospitals and guide reimbursement are challenging to create, implement, and interpret.

Washington State Provider Profiling

Increasingly, surgeons are faced with payment reform efforts and evolving financial incentives based on comparative effectiveness data to improve the quality of care, such as the Centers for Medicare and Medicaid Services (CMS) Meaningful Use requirements. The field of comparative effectiveness is a relatively new field that tries to answer the question "what works best," often in the context of real-world scenarios instead of controlled laboratory results. CMS's Meaningful Use requirements was a system of offering increased reimbursement to healthcare providers that had implemented robust Electronic Health Record (EHR) systems, another example of using reimbursement to guide clinical practice.

As state and federal agencies struggle to curb healthcare spending increases, they have pursued measures to ensure quality. For example, Washington State's Administrative Code (WAC 296-20-01010) establishes oversight for a network of providers approved to treat injured workers covered by the Washington State fund and self-insured employers. This policy excludes certain providers from providing care to injured workers covered by the fund, stating "it is the intent of the department, through authority granted by RCW 51.36.010 to protect workers from physical or psychiatric harm by identifying, and taking appropriate action, including removal of providers from the statewide network, when (a) there is harm; (b) there is a pattern of low quality care, and (c) the harm is related to the pattern of low quality care." This policy is potentially one of the more forceful policies of payer intervention into clinical practice to improve clinical outcomes.

According to WAC definitions, "low-quality care" includes practices "that have not been shown to be safe or effective, or for which it has been shown that the risks of harm exceed the benefits that can reasonably be expected, based on available peer-reviewed scientific studies ... or those that include repeated unsuccessful surgical or other invasive procedure." In lumbar surgery this arguably includes the discordant use of fusion to treat poorly supported indications such as disc herniation, disc degeneration, and spinal stenosis in the absence of spondylolisthesis – a policy similar to the Blue Cross Blue Shield of North Carolina policy highlighted earlier. In addition, greater "surgical invasiveness" in spine surgery, as measured by multilevel fusion, combined anterior-posterior surgical approaches, and use of stabilizing instrumentation, increases complications without consistent evidence of improved patient outcomes and therefore could be not covered under the WAC's administrative codes.

Under WAC, "harms" are defined as the "intended or unintended physical or psychiatric injury resulting from, or contributed to, health care services that result in the need for additional monitoring, treatment or hospitalization or that worsens the condition(s), increases disability, or causes death. Harm includes increased, chronic, or prolonged pain or decreased function." A Delphi survey previously conducted among Washington State surgeons established a consensus that repeated spine surgery, infection, new neurological deficit, and mortality were essential and relevant measures of harm in spine surgery [4].

Under this legislation, Washington State's Department of Labor and Industries, which manages the State's worker's compensation (WC) system, is seeking to identify surgeons who exhibit a pattern of low-quality care leading to surgical harms. The department's initial focus is on surgical treatment for common lumbar degenerative conditions, including disc degeneration, disc herniation, spinal stenosis, spondylolisthesis, and adult scoliosis. It might be more meaningful to benchmark outcomes against those previously reported by the SPORT trials, and others might be used as grounds to qualify or disqualify spinal surgeons for reimbursement under the WAC codes [13–15]. The motivation to develop a network of providers based on profiling surgical harms derives from empiric data showing that discretionary surgeon decision-making explains up to 50% of the surgeon-level variation in surgical complications and 30% of surgeon-level variation in reoperation rates [16]. Thus, the exclusion of surgeons with relatively higher rates of harms, coupled with a patient's informed choice of a provider, may substantially reduce rates of surgical harms, reduce costs, and, most importantly, improve patient outcomes and satisfaction. Additionally, measuring patient safety against referenced benchmarks can motivate surgeons to engage in quality improvement efforts.

Conclusions

Policymakers hope to combat the rising costs of healthcare by guiding reimbursement toward high-value care and in the process influence how providers treat their patients. These efforts have produced a variety of policy responses with differing levels of success, as well as fostered a field of research that analyzes medical care from a population level. Back pain management is one area where there is a continual focus due to a high population prevalence of back pain, increasing rates of spine surgery, and the associated increases in costs and complications [17]. As reimbursement focuses on quality and patient outcome measures, it is essential to understand how these measures are created, implemented, and collected, as well as how providers respond to these incentives. The implementation of innovative policy and rigorous real-world analysis of these policies are imperative steps toward reducing the overutilization of spinal care and fairly reimbursing providers who perform safe, effective, and timely interventions.

References

1. Martin BI, et al. Effects of a commercial insurance policy restriction on lumbar fusion in North Carolina and the implications for national adoption. Spine (Phila Pa 1976). 2015;41:647.
2. Martin BI, et al. Indications for spine surgery: validation of an administrative coding algorithm to classify degenerative diagnoses. Spine (Phila Pa 1976). 2014;39(9):769–79.
3. Kazberouk A, et al. Validation of an administrative coding algorithm for classifying surgical indication and operative features of spine surgery. Spine (Phila Pa 1976). 2015;40(2):114–20.
4. Mirza SK, et al. Developing a toolkit for comparing safety in spine surgery. Instr Course Lect. 2014;63:271–86.
5. Mirza SK, et al. Development of an index to characterize the "invasiveness" of spine surgery: validation by comparison to blood loss and operative time. Spine (Phila Pa 1976). 2008;33(24):2651–2661; discussion 2662.
6. Martin B, Mirza SK, Spina N, Spiker WR, Lawrence B, Brodke DS. Trends in lumbar fusion procedure rates and associated hospital costs for degenerative spinal diseases in the United States, 2004-2015. Spine (Phila Pa 1976). 2018;44:369.
7. Martin BI, et al. How do coverage policies influence practice patterns, safety, and cost of initial lumbar fusion surgery? A population-based comparison of workers' compensation systems. Spine J. 2014;14(7):1237–46.
8. Martin BI, Lurie JD, Farrokhi FR, McGuire KJ, Mirza SK. Early effects of medicare's bundled payment for care improvement program for lumbar fusion. Spine (Phila Pa 1976). 2018;43(10):705–11.
9. Martin BI, Lurie JD, Tosteson AN, Deyo RA, Farrokhi FR, Mirza SK. Use of bone morphogenetic protein among patients undergoing fusion for degenerative diagnoses in the United States, 2002 to 2012. Spine J. 2015;15(4):692–9.
10. https://www.medicare.gov/hospitalcompare/search.html.
11. Ganduglia CM, Zezza M, Smith JD, John SD, Franzini L. Effect of public reporting on MR imaging use for low back pain. Radiology. 2015;276(1):175–83.
12. Martin BI, Jarvik JG. The medicare outpatient imaging efficiency measure for low back pain ("OP-8"). Radiology. 2015;276(1):1–2.
13. Weinstein JN, Lurie JD, Tosteson TD, Hanscom B, Tosteson AN, Blood EA, Birkmeyer NJ, Hilibrand AS, Herkowitz H, Cammisa FP, Albert TJ, Emery SE, Lenke LG, Abdu WA, Longley M, Errico TJ, Hu SS. Surgical versus nonsurgical treatment for lumbar degenerative spondylolisthesis. N Engl J Med. 2007;356(22):2257–70.
14. Weinstein JN, Tosteson TD, Lurie JD, Tosteson AN, Blood E, Hanscom B, Herkowitz H, Cammisa F, Albert T, Boden SD, Hilibrand A, Goldberg H, Berven S, An H, SPORT Investigators. Surgical versus nonsurgical therapy for lumbar spinal stenosis. N Engl J Med. 2008;358(8):794–810.

15. Ong KL, Auerbach JD, Lau E, Schmier J, Ochoa JA. Perioperative outcomes, complications, and costs associated with lumbar spinal fusion in older patients with spinal stenosis and spondylolisthesis. Neurosurg Focus. 2014;36(6):E5.
16. Martin BI, Mirza SK, Franklin GM, Lurie JD, MacKenzie TA, Deyo RA. Hospital and surgeon variation in complications and repeat surgery following incident lumbar fusion for common degenerative diagnoses. Health Serv Res. 2013;48(1):1–25.
17. Martin BI, et al. Expenditures and health status among adults with back and neck problems. JAMA. 2008;299(6):656–64.

The Bree Collaborative Bundle for Lumbar Fusion: Evolution of a Community Standard for Quality

3

Andrew S. Friedman
and Robert S. Mecklenburg

Lumbar fusion is the treatment of choice when neurological function is threatened by spinal instability due to trauma, tumor, infection, or congenital anomalies. The benefits of this procedure are much less certain, however, when lumbar fusion is applied to non-urgent conditions such as chronic back pain without neurologic findings. For this large cohort of patients, high and variable charges, high complication rates, and escalating utilization rate across the United States – coupled with uncertain benefits – have provoked increased scrutiny from purchasers and the provider community alike. The current state is not only costly for purchasers and sometimes dangerous for patients, but it is harmful to the

A. S. Friedman (✉)
Neuroscience Institute, Virginia Mason Medical Center, Seattle, WA, USA

Department of Physical Medicine and Rehabilitation, Virginia Mason Medical Center, Seattle, WA, USA
e-mail: Andrew.Friedman@virginiamason.org

R. S. Mecklenburg
Center for Healthcare Solutions, Department of Medicine, Virginia Mason Hospital and Seattle Medical Center, Seattle, WA, USA

© Springer Nature Switzerland AG 2020   39
R. K. Sethi et al. (eds.), *Value-Based Approaches to Spine Care*,
https://doi.org/10.1007/978-3-030-31946-5_3

credibility of those providers working to improve the safety, appropriateness, reliability, effectiveness, and affordability of lumbar surgical techniques.

In this chapter we will describe efforts over the last 14 years to improve our approach to lumbar fusion and to ensure that this procedure remains a credible, valuable, and sustainable alternative for those patients likely to receive benefit.

Identifying and Managing Uncomplicated Back Pain: The Spine Clinic

The foundation of ensuring appropriate utilization of lumbar surgery and lumbar fusion in particular is proper patient selection. Systems to promptly identify patients with uncomplicated back pain and early implementation of appropriate non-surgical care have been shown to provide high levels of patient satisfaction and reduction in cost compared to usual care. Recent studies have also shown early conservative care to lower rates of opioid utilization [1]. This approach serves to avoid unnecessary diagnostic procedures and surgery in many patients who have access to such care. Our experience indicates that the preferred initial contact with the health-care system for patients with non-emergent back pain should be with non-surgical spine specialists. Specifically in our institution, initial specialty contact with physiatrists and physical therapists has proven to provide high levels of patient satisfaction and outcomes for the majority of patients with lumbar spine disorders. In addition to these direct benefits, the utilization of non-surgical specialists for initial care reduces unnecessary surgical consultations, improves access to surgeons for necessary consultations, and is associated with high "conversion rates" for appropriate spine surgery cases. At Virginia Mason, a method for separating patients who required surgical care from those who did not was developed in concert with the health benefits team at Starbucks.

Engagement with Employers and the Marketplace Collaborative Model

In 2004, major Seattle-based employers, including Starbucks, Costco, and King County, met with us to voice serious concerns regarding the high cost of health care at our institution and announce their intent to remove Virginia Mason from their network of providers [2]. As with many employers, care of spinal conditions was a major element of their annual spend. We began our work with employers by acknowledging our accountability for costly, low-value care.

Two years earlier, Virginia Mason Medical Center had adopted the Toyota Production System as a management method – a method focusing on the reduction of waste. As a result, we clearly understood both the magnitude of unnecessary care we were delivering and how to improve our performance. As an alternative to being excluded from the provider network, we offered the employers and their health plan, Aetna, the opportunity to reengineer health-care delivery to improve quality and affordability. The employers and Aetna accepted our invitation, and we launched the first "Marketplace Collaborative" in which employers bring their purchasing power directly to bear on improving the delivery of health care.

Our first task was to determine the list of health-care priorities for employers. Employers gave us access to their claims data. Evaluation of these data, including both direct payment and loss of productivity, revealed the greatest cost to employers – back pain – high on the list of the ten most costly conditions for Starbucks and their colleagues. This list became our agenda, with back pain as our first priority.

In order to establish design principles for management of back pain, the second task for our collaborative was to understand quality from the perspective of the employer/purchaser. The group had no difficulty in declaring the "purchasing specs" by which they wished to procure health care. They listed five requirements:

1. Evidence-based medicine: care that works
2. 100% customer satisfaction: the patient care experience
3. Same-day access
4. Rapid return to function
5. Affordable price for buyer and seller

When we mapped the typical patient pathway for back pain through Virginia Mason and showed the results to Starbucks, we were embarrassed that the process was characterized by substantial waits and delays, frequent needless consultations and imaging, and high variation among providers. This was our baseline. Within 3 months, we redesigned our model for care of back pain with Starbucks and Aetna, creating the "Spine Clinic" according to the five design specifications. To do so, we reviewed medical literature to identify evidence-based practice, used Lean methodology to eliminate non-value content from our current practice and to standardize provider practice, and concentrated on cost accounting to monitor finances for both the employer and Virginia Mason.

Redesigning the Care Pathway for Uncomplicated Back Pain

The initial process step in the Spine Clinic model is to separate patients into three categories: acute uncomplicated back pain, chronic or complex back pain, and acute complicated back pain which requires urgent or emergent care. This "triage" function is accomplished in a telephone-based intake process that generates a numerical score based on a set of questions. This task requires a 10-minute interview by our telephone team. Patients with "red flags" are immediately identified and referred to the emergency room or to a same-day appointment to an on-call spine surgeon. Patients with chronic complex back pain were referred to a physiatry consultation. The 80% of patients who have no symptoms to indicate a threatening abnormality or complex history are seen by physical therapist within one business day.

At the same-day 60-minute appointment, a physical therapist reviews the patient's history, performs a physical exam, and formulates a working plan. A physiatrist briefly joins the therapist and patient to review findings and confirm the plan, order any needed studies or medications, and provide additional reassurance and support. Opioids are used rarely and for only very short duration. Active physical therapy commences at the same office visit, usually including strengthening exercises, activity modification, and graduated activity plans. Important elements of this approach are establishing a working rehabilitation diagnosis and a collaborative plan among patient, physician, and therapist. The patient is provided with a home regimen. Return office visits are arranged – usually with the therapist or by telephone.

If the patient fails to improve promptly, we arrange imaging, additional studies, and a return visit with the physiatrist or specialty consultant or other interventions. To prevent unnecessary imaging in primary care, we installed a "mistake-proofing" tool in the scheduling process for a lumbar MRI, requiring the provider to check one of the evidence-based indications for the study. The alternative was to call the physiatrist on call to discuss the rationale for the test or arrange for a spine clinic visit.

Improved Quality and Timeliness of Care for Uncomplicated Back Pain

Since 2005, we have used refined versions of this basic model to manage over 30,000 patients. When we studied the effect of the Spine Clinic, we found that applying evidence-based decision rules reduced our utilization of lumbar MRI by 23.4% (Fig. 3.1) [3]. The resulting low "denial rate" with health plans led to exemptions from preauthorization. When the performance of the Spine Clinic was compared to local competitors, days of work loss were less (4.3 days vs. 8.8 days), with half the physical therapy visits (4.4 visits vs. 8.8 visits) [4]. The Spine Clinic also achieved high patient satisfaction ratings. An unpublished internal survey of 100 consecutive patients revealed a satisfaction rating of 4.9 out of 5.0.

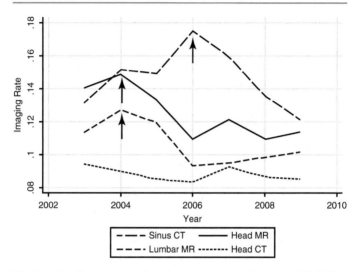

Fig. 3.1 Imaging rates vs. time for patients with disease-specific billing codes from a single regional payer. Arrows indicate the year before the intervention. (The full description of the intervention was provided by Blackmore et al. [3]. Figure shared with permission)

Financial Consequences for Providers

Our design specifications for the Spine Clinic required financial sustainability for providers as well as employers. One of the major challenges we faced in improving efficiency of care for patients requiring either surgical or non-surgical care for back pain is the fee-for-service payment methodology used by health plans. Eliminating non-value-added care results in a prompt reduction in revenue stream by providers and creates the threat of a business model that is non-sustainable. We successfully addressed this situation in the following ways:

1. "Skill/task alignment." The hourly cost of providing care with a physical therapist is 50% that of a non-proceduralist physician and 25% that of a spine surgeon. Our cost of producing care for uncomplicated back pain dropped dramatically with

the Spine Clinic model and illustrated the general principle that financial sustainability for providers will depend on lowering cost of production rather than attempting to either extract higher reimbursement rates from purchasers or deliver increased volumes of low-value care. The ability to leverage a team of providers – that includes lower-cost practitioners – coupled with the ability to rapidly escalate care to a higher level of expertise, allows for cost reduction and increased face-to-face time for patients without limiting diagnostic expertise or treatment options.

2. Increased throughput. The Spine Clinic model allowed us to quadruple patient volume by reducing waits and delays within the care process for providers. Office visits were efficient and predictable, and the triage method reduced inappropriate and complicated "surprises" in the schedule of physical therapists and physicians.

3. Payer mix. In general terms, employer contracts pay providers more than Medicare and much more than Medicaid. In co-designing care with employers according to their standards, providers gain a relationship based on value that can lead to preferential referral or even exclusive contracts. Regardless of reimbursement model, the efficient Spine Clinic model either maximizes margin or reduces financial losses

4. "Downstream revenue." The increased throughput of the Spine Clinic uncovers many more patients with a bona fide need for imaging or surgery. The Spine Clinic refers patients to spine surgeons that are strong surgical candidates. Spine surgeons spend much less time screening patients to identify surgical candidates. As a related example, when we initiated a similar approach for patients with breast nodules, the breast surgeon was sent only those patients requiring surgery. The "conversion rate" of breast surgeon office visits increased dramatically, and the productivity of the spine surgeon increased over 30% [5].

5. "Direct contracting." A spine clinic, taken as a financial "cost center," will have a positive margin only if reimbursement exceeds cost of production. With our Spine Clinic, Starbucks – a self-funded employer – paid less for higher

quality. But when we eliminated unnecessary imaging, consultations, and office visits, Virginia Mason Medical Center was projected to have a negative margin due to the fact that our contract with the health plan paid less for physical therapy than it cost to produce a physical therapy visit. In the Marketplace Collaborative model, finances are transparent, and Starbucks quickly realized that the much-improved model was not sustainable for Virginia Mason Medical Center. Starbucks instructed Aetna to increase the reimbursement rate for physical therapy to create a positive margin for Virginia Mason Medical Center while ensuring savings for Starbucks [2]. This was our first experience with "direct contracting" with an employer where providers and employers not only set quality standards but also set a price that is fair to each. Setting reimbursement rates directly with the employer was foreshadowing of formal direct contracting for lumbar fusion.

Lessons Learned from Starbucks, the Marketplace Collaborative, and Spine Clinic

Our experience in developing the Spine Clinic was the foundation for the subsequent development of a sustainable model for lumbar fusion. We learned that:

1. It is desirable to begin by separating patients requiring surgery from those that do not. This can be facilitated by a scheduling tool administered by telephone prior to the first visit.
2. Patients with uncomplicated back pain are best treated by same-day access to physical therapy and a non-surgical provider with training in back pain. This approach provides the best care for patients, helps to avoid unnecessary surgery and imaging, and ensures that surgeons are deployed in performing surgery.
3. Design of patient care pathways is efficient and effective when providers interact directly with employers rather than health plans or other middlemen.

4. Self-insured employers, when informed and empowered in the Marketplace Collaborative model, are motivated to ensure a positive financial margin for providers that are providing prompt, reliable, value-added care. Collaborating directly with employers, in a format that encourages mutual support and accountability, engages employers with value-based purchasing with their medical center. Further, collaboration with employers provides encouragement to move beyond health care dominated by the business practice of health plans.

5. Improving appropriate non-surgical management of patients at a population level can increase market share and surgical volumes.

Replicating the Spine Clinic Model

Our success with the Spine Clinic model attracted national attention, but many expressed reservations that this approach was highly contingent on the culture, integrated structure, and the Lean methodology unique to Virginia Mason Medical Center. In 2009, we had the opportunity to test the hypothesis that this method could be implemented by other providers in other markets. Intel requested assistance from VM in evaluating the option of implementing the Spine Clinic in their Portland, Oregon market. Their claims data also indicated that back pain was on their short list of medical conditions most prevalent and costly for their workforce. Intel accepted the five quality indicators and recruited three provider groups and Cigna to participate in their collaborative. Virginia Mason providers presented the Spine Clinic model to the Oregon colleagues who accepted the method with minor modifications. A detailed work plan was developed and implemented based on Lean methodology. At the end of a year, data collected by Intel indicated that providers had met each of the five quality indicators with close to zero defects, saving Intel 24% in direct cost (Table 3.1) and reducing average duration of treatment from 52 days to 22 days (Fig. 3.2). Provider groups improved their finances by millions of dollars. With Intel, we published the results of this project in the Harvard Business Review [6].

Table 3.1 Costs of treating a condition was one of five metrics selected by Healthcare Marketplace Collaborative (HMC) to measure progress

Success measures	Lower back pain	Shoulder, knee, and hip pain	Headache	Breast problems	Upper respiratory illness	Diabetes	Screening
Same-day access	93%	86%	100%	26%	100%	100%	100%
Patient satisfaction	98%	98%	92%	94%	100%	96%	96%
Evidence-based medicine	92%	81%	N/A	100%	N/A	N/A	N/A
Rapid return to function	99%	97%	N/A	42%	N/A	N/A	N/A
Savings in direct costs	23.5%	37.7%	49.1%	N/A	N/A	N/A	N/A
Initiated	2010	2010	2011	2012	2012	2013	2012
Duration	35 mos.	35 mos.	24 mos.	38 mos.	18 mos.	10 mos.	14 mos.
No. of patients	499	343	657	86	111	47	151

From American Hospital Association and Irving Levin Associates. Reprinted with permission from "Health Care Needs Real Competition" by Leemore S. Dafny and Thomas H. Lee. Harvard Business Review, December 2016. Copyright 2016 by Harvard Business Publishing; all rights reserved

Note the value streams were uncomplicated back pain; uncomplicated shoulder, knee, and hip pain; uncomplicated headaches (migraines); breast problems (lumps, pain, redness, discharge); uncomplicated upper respiratory illness; diabetes; screening for influenza and pneumonia immunizations and to detect illnesses such as diabetes, high blood pressure, and colon and breast cancer

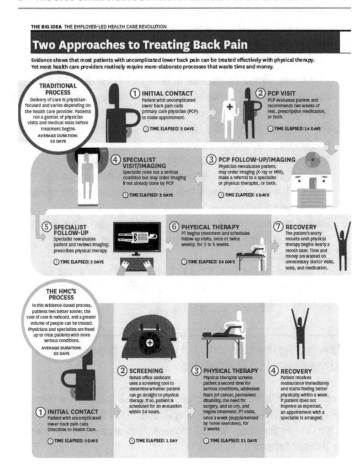

Fig. 3.2 Two approaches to treating spinal pain. (From American Hospital Association and Irving Levin Associates. Reprinted with permission from "Health Care Needs Real Competition" by Leemore S. Dafny and Thomas H. Lee. Harvard Business Review, December 2016. Copyright 2016 by Harvard Business Publishing; all rights reserved)

Lessons Learned from Intel's Collaborative and the Spine Clinic

1. The Spine Clinic model and delivery of the five quality specifications can be successfully replicated by providers and employers outside Seattle and Virginia Mason Medical Center. Of note, a substantial proportion of providers were not employed in an integrated system.
2. Direct oversight by the employer required sharing of information on process improvement across provider groups that quickly began to collaborate and outdistance their competitors in delivering value.
3. Direct communication between providers and employer was efficient and effective. The contribution of the health plan became secondary.
4. At the end of the project, Intel proceeded with using the five quality indicators for direct contracting with providers in another market [7].

Beyond Spine Clinic: Contributions from Spine Surgery and Orthopedics

As the Spine Clinic model for uncomplicated back pain was being refined, two developments in surgical sections at Virginia Mason helped to set the stage for subsequent development of the bundle for lumbar fusion:

1. In 2010, the section of orthopedic surgery undertook process improvements to standardize their approach to total joint replacement. The section divided the patient care pathway into four discrete elements: recognizing which patients required joint replacement, preparing the patient for surgery, providing standardized best practice surgery, and ensuring rapid return to function. This four-cycle model led to major improvements in joint replacement and was later adapted to lumbar fusion.

2. In 2009, a patient undergoing multilevel deformity correction died during surgery. This event led to suspension of such surgery while a root cause analysis was performed. A number of contributing factors were identified, including inefficient transfer of information within the operative team, lack of a systematic method for preoperative planning, and the unreasonable task of a single attending surgeon performing a lengthy and complicated procedure. A preoperative multidisciplinary conference, improved communication methods for managing transfusion, and a second attending surgeon were designed to correct deficiencies. These methods were implemented as multilevel spinal fusion was resumed. The results were a striking reduction in complication rate for complex spine surgery [8]. These elements informed subsequent standards for all lumbar fusion procedures.

The Robert Bree Collaborative: Putting It All Together

In 2011, the legislature of the state of Washington passed a bill creating a multi-stakeholder collaborative, the Robert Bree Collaborative (Bree), to improve quality, safety, and affordability of health care. The Governor appointed 22 members, representing employers, providers, health plans, and quality organizations. Every year Bree chooses three priority conditions and then convenes a work group to produce explicit voluntary state standards for care delivery. All meetings are public and all documents produced by the work group are in the public domain. In 2011, one of the priority topics selected by Bree was uncomplicated back pain. Recommendations released in 2013 were similar to Virginia Mason's Spine Clinic. In 2014, Bree extended its agenda related to spine conditions by commissioning a work group to create a bundled payment model for lumbar fusion. The lumbar fusion bundle was updated in 2018. Bree extended its agenda related to spine conditions by creating a bundled payment model for lumbar fusion in 2014. A 2018 update of the bundle contained no major changes.

The strategic importance of Bree in health-care reform is to create a single state-wide standard for quality to form the foundation for the production, purchasing, and payment of health care.

Bree Collaborative Work Group on Lumbar Fusion

The work group on lumbar fusion included spine surgeons, physiatrists, medical center administrators, large employers, health plans, a quality organization, and a patient advocate. The group met monthly for a year to develop the product. Among the contributions from stakeholders was the four-cycle model Virginia Mason Medical Center had developed for joint replacement. Bree renamed these cycles appropriateness, fitness for surgery, evidence-based surgery, and rapid return to function. The bundle was created by the work group by first proposing elements for each cycle and then applying the tools of evidence-based medicine to either validate or eliminate them. The work group added quality metrics resembling the five purchase specs previously tested by employers. Finally, the work group added a warranty against avoidable readmissions. Drafts produced by the work group were reviewed and approved by the full Bree Collaborative every few months and then posted on the Bree website for public comment. The work group met to adjust the bundle based on public comment. After a final approval by the full collaborative, the document was signed by the Administrator of Washington State's Health Care Authority as a voluntary standard for providers, employers, health plans, or others that could be used for care delivery, purchasing, and payment. Bree does not produce, purchase, or pay for health care.

The bundle for lumbar fusion included a number of innovations designed to disrupt the current state. These included an evidence table posted in the public domain, shared decision-making, a multidisciplinary conference chaired by a physiatrist to determine whether surgical or non-surgical care is recommended, market-relevant quality metrics reported to employer by provider every 3 months, and the warranty against avoidable complications. The structure of the bundle was designed to facilitate direct contracting between providers and employers. We will now review these elements in further detail.

The Evidence Table

The work group understood that one of the fundamental barriers to safety, quality, and affordability was opinion-based variation in practice. The group therefore sought to reinforce each of the quality standards within the four-cycle model with best available medical evidence. A research librarian collaborated with the work group to search medical literature on each recommendation included in the bundle. For appraisal of citations, the work group adopted the Strength of Recommendation Taxonomy [9]. Two physicians credentialed in evidence appraisal reviewed each citation to reach accord on grading of each research paper. Hundreds of citations were reviewed and appraised. The evidence table was made available in the public domain for further critique. Over 100 citations support the 4 cycles of the bundle. Medical literature was systematically reviewed on a 3-year cycle, sooner if important new findings came to light. At the conclusion of the work group's efforts, the following elements were included in evidence-based standards within the four cycles. Details are included in the official bundle document that can be located at http://www.breecollaborative.org/topic-areas/apm/.

Cycle One: Standards for Appropriateness for Lumbar Fusion

The appropriateness cycle includes five requirements:

1. Specification of the patient's degree of functional impairment using the PROMIS-10 survey and the Oswestry Disability Index.
2. Documentation of imaging findings confirming lumbar instability that correlate with the patient's symptoms and signs.

3. Documentation of at least 3 months of structured non-surgical therapy delivered by a collaborative team.
4. Documentation of severe disability unresponsive to non-surgical therapy, documentation of persistent disability after the course of a non-surgical care. This section also includes formal consultation with collaborative team led by a designated physician (preferably a physiatrist) to confirm appropriateness, adequacy, completeness, and active participation in non-surgical therapy and need for lumbar fusion
5. Shared decision-making.

Cycle Two: Fitness for Surgery

This cycle includes three general requirements:

1. Requirements for patient safety. This section includes 12 specific patient safety requirements that include a BMI less than 40, avoidance of nicotine for at least 4 weeks preoperatively, management of any chronic opioid use, a hemoglobin A1C of less than 8% in patients with diabetes, and other requirements as listed on the Bree website.
2. Patient engagement. These requirements include selection of a personal care partner (lay care partner), participation in end-of-life planning, and agreement to participate in the surgical registry.
3. Documentation of optimal preparation for surgery that includes relevant consultations and a screen for risk factors for delirium.

Cycle Three: Best Practice Surgery

This cycle includes six requirements for optimal surgery including:

1. Multimodal anesthesia and minimization of the use of opioids
2. Measures to avoid infection
3. Measures to avoid bleeding and low blood pressure

4. Measures to avoid deep venous thrombosis and pulmonary embolism
5. Measures to avoid hyperglycemia
6. Standards for the use of bone morphogenetic protein
7. Annual surgical volume of 30 fusions per surgeon, 60 fusions per facility, and participation in a spine surgery registry

Cycle Four: Rapid Return to Function

This cycle includes four requirements:

1. A standard process for postoperative care
2. Use of a standardized facility discharge process aligned with Washington State Hospital Association (WSHA) toolkit
3. Arrangement of home health services if needed
4. Scheduling of follow-up appointments that include continued surveillance of nicotine cessation when applicable

The Multidisciplinary Conference

Each patient who is a candidate for lumbar fusion is presented at the weekly multidisciplinary conference. Multiple spine surgeons, physiatrists, physical therapists, members of the anesthesia pain service, and operational leaders attend the conference with others as needed. A physiatrist chairs this conference. Each patient's history and physical examination is reviewed, and assessment of completion of cycles one and two are displayed on a purpose-built computerized page. The group discusses and debates risks, benefits, and alternatives. A treatment plan is determined by the group. The physiatrist records proceedings and recommendations of the conference in the medical record, and a member of the multidisciplinary team reviews this recommendation with the patient.

If a patient does not meet appropriateness or safety standards, the team develops a plan to prepare the patient for surgery or, if surgery is inappropriate, recommends a non-surgical course of care.

The Personal Care Partner

The patient designates a competent care partner who accompanies them through the entire care process, serving as an advocate to facilitate communication and to assist the patient, particularly following hospital discharge. If patient's residence is distant from the medical center, the care partner travels with the patient. If patient cannot or will not designate a care partner, the surgical team should discuss how to best support the patient post-surgery and document this plan in the medical record.

Quality Measures

Quality measures were determined with major input from employers. Unlike many claims-based processes, these market-relevant measures address issues of high importance to both patients and employers. The specific requirements are reported quarterly by the provider directly to the employer and include the following specifics:

1. Appropriateness. The proportion of patients undergoing lumbar fusion that have participated in shared decision-making
2. Evidence-based surgery. The proportion of patients in which the surgical team delivered all elements of best practice surgery as outlined in cycle three
3. Rapid return to function. The proportion of patients who completed patient required reported outcome measures following surgery
4. Patient care experience. The proportion of patients surveyed using HCAHPS or OAS CAHPS
5. Patient safety and affordability. The 30-day all-cause readmission rate and readmission rate following lumbar fusion surgery for any of the avoidable hospitalizations specified in the warranty

The Warranty Against Avoidable Remissions

Bree's work group for lumbar fusion used a study commissioned by CMS for total joint replacement as the basis for its warranty [10]. The CMS study included both complications that could be attributable to surgery and the risk windows during which accountability for complications is in effect. If a patient is readmitted to the hospital where the surgery was performed within the specified risk window and with one of the avoidable complications, no additional charges can be required of the purchaser.

The risk windows and surgical complications are as follows:

1. 7 days following hospital discharge: acute myocardial infarction, pneumonia, sepsis/septicemia
2. 30 days following hospital discharge: pulmonary embolism, surgical site bleeding, superficial surgical site infection
3. 90 days following hospital discharge: deep surgical site infection that may involve the implant, mechanical complications

Definitions and code sets associated with these applications are recorded on the Bree website.

Response of Health-Care Stakeholders to Surgical Bundles

The Bree Collaborative has produced four surgical bundles: total joint replacement, lumbar fusion, coronary artery bypass grafting, and bariatric surgery. The following comments apply to Bree Collaborative bundles for total joint replacement, completed in 2013, and the lumbar fusion bundle, completed in 2014.

Employers

Several large purchasers have embraced the bundled payment model as an approach to value-based purchasing, notably CMS, Walmart, and the Washington State Health Care Authority (HCA). Our experience with the HCA has been most instructive. The HCA began direct contracting with providers using Bree's bundle for total joint replacement, adding a fixed-price, prospective payment feature and direct contracting between employer and provider.

HCA's most disruptive innovation was to use a request for proposals, sent to solicit providers that could deliver care according to the bundle's quality specifications. This approach gives the employer a high degree of control over the quality of their providers, in marked contrast to networks created by health plans without clear regard to market-relevant quality. The transparent, evidence-based bundle allows employers to know exactly what they are purchasing. The prospective, fixed-payment feature and warranty allows them to know exactly how much they will pay, and the quality measures allow them to determine if the care improved the function of their employee. The HCA recently reported their results for the joint replacement bundle in the *New England Journal of Medicine Catalyst* [11]. In short, compared to their control group, costs were less and quality improved. Patient satisfaction was excellent. Direct contracting using the Bree bundle eliminates much of the administrative cost of health-care middlemen, particularly health plans and their business practices that include preauthorization, opaque reimbursement models in a fee-for-service format, denials, appeals, and complex benefit options. In our view, the main barrier for smaller employers to enter the bundle market is their dependence on health plans.

Health Plans

Health plans have been slow to embrace Bree bundles that "disintermediate" them, allowing direct contracting, collaboration, and contracting between employers and providers. Direct contracting means that health plans lose control over setting reimbursement rates. And they lose control over the practice of medicine through preauthorization and denials. Fee-for-service medicine can be eliminated as a payment methodology.

Providers

Bree bundles set a high-quality bar for providers, requiring a transition from opinion-based, provider-specified care to evidence-informed, systems-based standardized care. Progressive providers in integrated medical centers are advantaged in meeting Bree standards. When provider groups, such as Virginia Mason Medical Center, meet these standards and win contracts through an RFP process, they gain market share – often against large, consolidated competitors. This has been our experience.

Providers must be ready for several challenges. The administrative cost of implementing a bundle program must attract sufficient patients and a favorable reimbursement rate to result in a positive margin. In addition, applying Bree standards for appropriateness and fitness for lumbar fusion surgery indicated that 58% of patients referred to Virginia Mason for this procedure did not meet these fundamental requirements [12], an obvious loss of revenue. The increase in market share at a favorable rate offset these losses at Virginia Mason and has allowed us to continue our progress in collaborating with employers in value-based purchasing.

Summary

In this chapter we have reviewed Virginia Mason's approach to delivering spine care that ensures high quality for patients, affordability for employers, and both clinical and financial success for providers. Our approach requires integration of care; application of evidence-informed, systems-based care pathways; multidisciplinary decision-making; market-relevant measures of performance; and close collaboration with employers with value-based contracting. Our success with these models at Virginia Mason Medical Center presents an opportunity for elite spine care centers to assume a leadership position in market-based health-care reform.

References

1. Sun E, Moshfegh J, Rishel CA, Cook CE, Goode AP, George SZ. Association of early physical therapy with long-term opioid use among opioid-naive patients with musculoskeletal pain. JAMA Netw Open. 2018;1(8):e185909-e.
2. Fuhrmans V. A novel plan helps hospital wean itself off pricey tests. Wall Street J. 2007;12:78–92.
3. Blackmore CC, Mecklenburg RS, Kaplan GS. Effectiveness of clinical decision support in controlling inappropriate imaging. J Am Coll Radiol. 2011;8(1):19–25.
4. Lee TH, Porter M. The strategy that will fix healthcare. Boston: Harvard Business Review; 2013.
5. Blackmore CC, Edwards JW, Searles C, Wechter D, Mecklenburg R, Kaplan GS. Nurse practitioner–staffed clinic at Virginia Mason improves care and lowers costs for women with benign breast conditions. Health Aff. 2013;32(1):20–6.
6. McDonald PA, Mecklenburg RS, Martin LA. The employer-led health care revolution. Harv Bus Rev. 2015;93(7-8):38–50, 133.
7. Care C. Employer-led innovation for healthcare delivery and payment reform: Intel Corporation and Presbyterian Healthcare Services.
8. Sethi RK, Pong RP, Leveque J-C, Dean TC, Olivar SJ, Rupp SM. The Seattle Spine Team approach to adult deformity surgery: a systems-based approach to perioperative care and subsequent reduction in perioperative complication rates. Spine Deform. 2014;2(2):95–103.
9. Ebell MH, Siwek J, Weiss BD, Woolf SH, Susman J, Ewigman B, et al. Strength of recommendation taxonomy (SORT): a patient-centered approach to grading evidence in the medical literature. J Am Board Fam Pract. 2004;17(1):59–67.
10. Robert Bree Collaborative warranty for elective total knee & total hip replacement surgery Washington State 2013. Available from: http://www.breecollaborative.org/wp-content/uploads/bree_warranty_tkr_thr.pdf.
11. Peterson M, Rolph S. Improving care by redesigning payment. NEJM Catalyst. 2018.
12. Yanamadala V, Kim Y, Buchlak QD, Wright AK, Babington J, Friedman A, et al. Multidisciplinary evaluation leads to the decreased utilization of lumbar spine fusion: an observational cohort pilot study. Spine. 2017;42(17):E1016–E23.

Multidisciplinary Evaluation Improves the Value of Lumbar Spine Care

4

Vijay Yanamadala, Anna K. Wright, Andrew S. Friedman, Reza Yassari, Andrew I. Gitkind, Robert S. Mecklenburg, and Rajiv K. Sethi

---

V. Yanamadala
Department of Neurosurgery, Montefiore Medical Center
and Albert Einstein College of Medicine, The Bronx, NY, USA

Center for Surgical Optimization, Leo M. Davidoff Department
of Neurosurgery, Montefiore Medical Center, The Bronx, NY, USA

A. K. Wright (✉)
Neuroscience Institute, Virginia Mason Medical Center,
Seattle, WA, USA
e-mail: Anna.Wright@virginiamason.org

A. S. Friedman
Neuroscience Institute, Virginia Mason Medical Center,
Seattle, WA, USA

Department of Physical Medicine and Rehabilitation,
Virginia Mason Medical Center, Seattle, WA, USA

R. Yassari
Department of Neurosurgery, Montefiore Medical Center
and Albert Einstein College of Medicine, The Bronx, NY, USA

A. I. Gitkind
Division of Interventional Spine, Department of Rehabilitation
Medicine, Montefiore Medical Center, Albert Einstein College
of Medicine, The Bronx, NY, USA

© Springer Nature Switzerland AG 2020
R. K. Sethi et al. (eds.), *Value-Based Approaches to Spine Care*,
https://doi.org/10.1007/978-3-030-31946-5_4

R. S. Mecklenburg
Center for Healthcare Solutions, Department of Medicine,
Virginia Mason Hospital and Seattle Medical Center, Seattle, WA, USA

R. K. Sethi
Neuroscience Institute, Departments of Neurosurgery Health Services,
Virginia Mason Medical Center, Seattle, WA, USA

The surgical treatment of degenerative spinal disease in the United States has increased tremendously in the past several decades. Nationwide Inpatient Sample (NIS) data reveals an eightfold increase in the rates of lumbar fusion for degenerative spondylosis between 1979 and 2012. Along with skyrocketing utilization rates, the total cost of spine surgery increased at the same rate between 1998 and 2008, far outpacing the cost increases associated with any other medical procedure. While lumbar spine surgery for spondylosis has been demonstrated to be effective in a randomized controlled trial setting for carefully selected patient populations, nationwide analyses have demonstrated that overall outcomes have largely stagnated and in some cases appear no better than nonoperative care. Importantly, the reasons for this dichotomous heterogeneity remain to be elucidated.

In the United States, management decisions for patients with degenerative spinal disease largely rest with the individual spine surgeon who typically makes all of the surgical and nonsurgical treatment decisions [1–3]. The virtues of shared decision-making for spinal disorders between surgeon and *patient* have been reported in a number of studies [4–8], and numerous decision support tools exist to ultimately make this process possible [9]. However, spine surgeons continue largely to practice without face-to-face communication with nonsurgical providers such as therapists, physiatrists, and interventionalists whose input can bring significantly different perspectives to patient care.

Virginia Mason Medical Center (VMMC) has been at the forefront of a multidisciplinary approach in adult deformity surgery [10], and other centers throughout the United States have also extolled the benefits of multidisciplinary care paradigms in treating complex spinal disorders [11]. The advantage of these multidisciplinary paradigms clearly extends to degenerative spine conditions, and centers around the country are now demonstrating that these approaches can reduce overutilization and inappropriate interventions.

The simplest of such approaches involve multidisciplinary care pathways, where different specialists develop standards and appropriateness criteria. The rates of surgical procedures and MRI utilization decrease after implementation of such multidisciplinary care pathways [12–14], without evidence of a decline in patient outcomes [15]. Many of these pathways revolve around medical triage of patients with spinal disorders, prior to seeing a surgeon. This is typically done by a physiatrist or another nonsurgical provider, which may include an internal medicine physician. Such pathways fundamentally alter the referral process. Concerns about overutilization of spine surgery have led to increasing pressure from payer groups to restrict spine surgery access and reimbursement [16]. These interventions can help build in the appropriateness and reverse this trend. However, the next step in the evolution of multidisciplinary spine care is true multidisciplinary decision-making.

Multidisciplinary Conferences

In November 2015, Virginia Mason Medical Center in Seattle, Washington, implemented a weekly multidisciplinary conference to review patients with lumbar degenerative spine conditions. Required attendees include members from physical medicine and rehabilitation, anesthesia pain, neurosurgery, orthopedic spine surgery, nursing, and physical therapy. We hypothesized that facilitating direct communication among local content experts in lumbar degenerative conditions may alter the treatment plan.

These multidisciplinary spine conferences are held every Tuesday morning at 7 AM and require a quorum of ten providers at minimum, including at least one provider from each of the following areas: physical medicine and rehabilitation (PM&R), the anesthesia pain service, neurosurgery and orthopedic spine surgery, nursing, and physical therapy. Each provider is given an equal voice and input in the decision-making process for each patient.

The patients reviewed in this multidisciplinary conference may present to any of the involved services, including neurosurgery, orthopedic spine surgery, PM&R, or the anesthesia pain service. The providers use the following selection criteria to determine the appropriateness of each patient for presentation at the spine conference:

1. Patients scheduled to undergo spine surgery involving up to five levels of fusion (patients who were scheduled to undergo more than five levels of fusion were presented separately in a complex spine multidisciplinary conference)
2. Patients who had been recommended up to five levels of spinal fusion at another institution and presented to a provider at Virginia Mason for a second opinion
3. Patients presenting with unusual spinal pathology that would, by the opinion of the primary presenting provider, benefit from a multidisciplinary discussion for diagnosis or treatment planning

The consulting physician presents patient's case at the conference and describes their assessment of the patient as well as any additional treatment recommendation made at other institutions. The entire team as a whole reviews imaging studies. After the group in attendance reaches a consensus opinion on how to proceed with the care of the patient, that recommendation is recorded in the patient's electronic medical record (EMR). The consulting physician then conveys the group's recommendations to the patient.

The multidisciplinary conference process was recently reviewed and published in a study by the multidisciplinary spine team from Virginia Mason Medical Center (VMMC). In this study, the records of consecutive patients who were presented at the multidisciplinary conference between November 2015 and November 2016 were reviewed. Patients who had been recommended a lumbar fusion procedure at an outside institution were further identified, and this group amounted to 100 consecutive patients of a total of 168 patients, as documented in outside consultation reports and confirmed by the patient at the time of initial consultation at VMMC [1].

The most common presenting diagnosis among patients who had been recommended for spinal fusion by an outside surgeon was spondylolisthesis (ten patients, 20%). Lumbar stenosis with claudication or radiculopathy was the second most common diagnosis (nine patients, 18%). Degenerative disc disease with axial back pain in the absence of radicular symptoms was the third most common diagnosis (five patients, 10%). Three patients (6%) had a diagnosis of symptomatic adjacent segment disease after prior fusion. Symptomatic pseudoarthrosis was the presenting diagnosis in two patients (4%). Work-up conducted as part of our multidisciplinary conference revealed misdiagnosis in two cases (4%) by the outside spine surgeon, with two cases of suspected lumbar radiculopathy identified as arising from degenerative hip changes.

Of these patients who had been recommended a lumbar fusion by an outside surgeon, only 58% had undergone any physical therapy; 70% had undergone a prior epidural steroid injection; 38% had undergone prior spine surgery at the site of proposed surgery or at an adjacent level. With regard to procedure type, 82% were recommended to undergo lumbar posterolateral fusion by an outside surgeon, while 16% were recommended a lumbar interbody fusion.

Of the 100 patients who had been recommended lumbar fusion at an outside institution, the multidisciplinary conference recommended 58% should not undergo immediate spine surgery ($\chi^2 = 26.6$; $p < 0.01$) as summarized in Fig. 4.1 and further depicted in Table 4.1. The patients (two patients, 4%) identified with hip pathology rather than lumbar radiculopathy were referred to a joint specialist for further evaluation and possible treatment. Ten patients (10%) were deemed currently inappropriate surgical candidates due to morbid obesity (BMI > 40). These patients were recommended to the VMMC bariatric medicine and surgery center for weight loss counseling. Ten patients (10%) were deemed inappropriate surgical candidates because they were active smokers at the time of consultation and were referred to the VMMC smoking cessation program with the acknowledgment that their case would be revisited should they successfully stop smoking with two documented negative urine cotinine checks. Twenty-two patients (22%) were deemed likely to benefit from additional

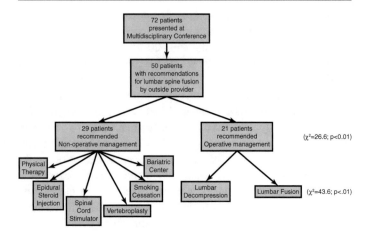

Fig. 4.1 Summary of patient selection, conference decision, and final treatment paradigm

Table 4.1 Number of patients deemed operative and nonoperative by the outside spine surgeon and the Virginia Mason Medical Center multidisciplinary spine conference

	Operative	Nonoperative
Outside surgeon	50	0
Conference	21	29

Of the 50 patients we identified for the study, the multidisciplinary conference recommended that 29 patients (58%) should not undergo any spine surgery ($\chi^2 = 26.6$; $p < 0.01$)

From Yanamadala et al. [1], with permission

physical therapy and were recommended PT prior to consideration of surgery. Six patients (6%) were deemed candidates for epidural steroid injection prior to surgical consideration, and two patients (2%) were deemed a candidate for vertebroplasty rather than surgery. Notably, the absence of physical therapy or ESI was not a contraindication for surgery, and eight patients (8%), all of

Table 4.2 The reasons for the recommendation of nonoperative management by the Virginia Mason Medical Center multidisciplinary spine conference

	Number of patients	Percentage
Misdiagnosis by outside surgeon	6	6%
Morbid obesity (BMI > 40)	10	10%
Active smoking	10	10%
Likely to benefit from additional physical therapy	22	22%
Likely to benefit from ESI	6	6%

From Yanamadala et al. [1], with permission

whom had spondylolisthesis, who had not had physical therapy previously were deemed surgical candidates as the physiatrists and physical therapists felt that they would not benefit from PT and would therefore be better served by surgical treatment. These rationales for recommending alternative management strategies are summarized in Table 4.2.

Of the 42 patients who underwent surgery, we found that 16 patients (38%) underwent a different procedure after multidisciplinary discussion than that previously recommended by the outside surgeon. Only 18 patients underwent lumbar posterolateral fusion without interbody, compared to 42 who had been recommended a lumbar posterolateral fusion by an outside surgeon ($\chi^2 = 43.6$; $p < .01$). Fourteen patients underwent lumbar interbody fusion compared to 16 who had been previously recommended the same ($\chi^2 = 0.79.6$; $p > .05$), and six patients who had been recommended lumbar fusion underwent simple decompressive procedures (laminectomy in four cases and foraminotomy in two cases; $\chi^2 = 5.37$; $p < .05$). These data are summarized in Figs. 4.2 and 4.3. We found a zero percent 30-day complication rate for the operative patients in this series.

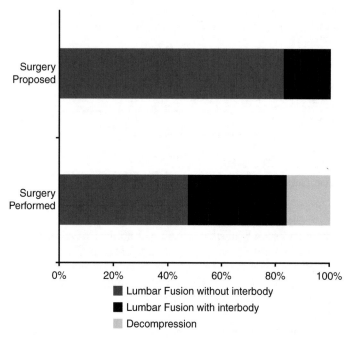

Fig. 4.2 The distribution of surgeries proposed by outside spine surgeons (surgery proposed) and the surgeries performed at Virginia Mason Medical Center on the operative patient group. Only nine patients underwent lumbar posterolateral fusion without interbody, compared to 42 who had been recommended a lumbar posterolateral fusion by an outside surgeon ($\chi^2 = 43.6$; $p < .01$). Seven patients underwent lumbar interbody fusion compared to eight who had been previously recommended the same ($\chi^2 = 0.79.6$; $p > .05$), and three patients who had been recommended lumbar fusion underwent simple decompressive procedures (laminectomy in two cases and foraminotomy in one case; $\chi^2 = 5.37$; $p < .05$). (From Yanamadala et al. [1], with permission)

While these initial results are promising, the outcomes of the patients who were not offered immediate surgery depend on the access to and adequacy of evidence-based and often multidisciplinary nonsurgical care which can often be a challenge in many communities in the United States.

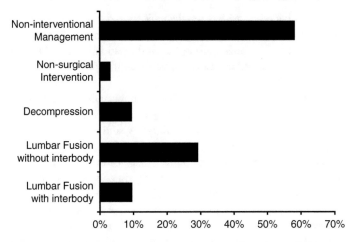

Fig. 4.3 Final management approach at Virginia Mason Medical Center for patients who were recommended a lumbar posterolateral fusion by an outside institution spine surgeon. (From Yanamadala et al. [1], with permission)

Multidisciplinary Clinics

Live multidisciplinary clinics are another way of implementing multidisciplinary strategies. Montefiore Medical Center (MMC), the University Hospital for Albert Einstein College of Medicine in New York City, has adopted a unique structure for the Montefiore Spine Center (MSC). A spine surgeon (neurosurgery or orthopedics), physiatrist, and interventionalist (from either an anesthesia or PM&R background) present simultaneously seeing patients and ultimately introducing patients to providers of other specialties as appropriate greatly facilitating multidisciplinary decision-making and multimodal treatment plans.

Starting in 2016, MSC has instituted this strategy to reduce variability in patient care throughout the medical center for patients with spine conditions. Patients are ultimately referred by outside providers to any of the providers in any of the departments including neurosurgery, orthopedic surgery, physiatry, anesthesia, and neurology.

These individual providers see the patients and discuss the individual cases with the other providers present in the clinic. This process generally involves both a discussion of the patient's clinical history and examination and review of the pertinent imaging.

Patient Example A patient with a lumbar disc herniation is referred to one of the physiatrists at MMC. The physiatrist sees the patient in clinic, obtains a full history, and reviews the imaging. She then engages the surgeon and interventionist present in clinic that day in a multidisciplinary discussion. They review the patient's history, including duration of pain and prior treatments, and deem the patient to be a potential surgical candidate. The consulting physiatrist then introduces the patient to the surgeon and interventionist. The three physicians, as a team, then discuss with the patient the nature of the pathology and treatment options including transforaminal epidural steroid injections or a microdiscectomy procedure. The patient decides that he would like surgery at this time and proceeds with surgery under the surgeons care the following week.

Initial data has suggested that this approach reduces lead time for patients who may benefit from multiple opinions, avoiding the referral and scheduling process for a second appointment, and also engages the providers in real-time multidisciplinary discussion involving the patient directly. Outcomes data are currently being collected by the center.

Discussion

It is ultimately undeniable that the utilization of spinal fusion in the United States has increased exponentially in the past few decades [17–23]. In parallel, the total cost of spine surgery increased 790% between 1998 and 2008, far outpacing any other medical procedure [24]. Between 1990 and 2000, the cost of total knee replacement increased a little over 200% [25], while dialysis costs have increased only 40% [26]. By definition, better value in spine care must involve either better outcomes or lower costs.

The ever-increasing cost and utilization of spine surgery without a concurrent increase in positive outcomes calls cost-effectiveness and quality of spine surgery into question. Value is often measured in quality-adjusted life years (QALYs) gained per dollar. Cost-effectiveness between interventions can be compared according to cost per QALY gained. Dialysis costs between $25,000 and $50,000 per QALY [27] and is considered the gold standard by which to benchmark other healthcare interventions. Total hip arthroplasty costs $4600 per QALY gained [28], while recent studies have shown that lumbar fusion may cost over $200,000 per QALY gained [29–31].

In the face of escalating costs, the value can be maintained by improving patient outcomes for a particular intervention. Unfortunately for lumbar fusion, numerous studies have shown that spinal fusion for low back pain is associated with stable or worse disability and return to work [32, 33] and that these outcomes may be even poorer in older patients and patients with more comorbidities [34], making its value proposition questionable. Lumbar fusion surgery does provide improvement for particular subsets of patients [35–42], and therefore the challenge lies in distinguishing those patients who are likely to see improvement after operative treatment from those who are better served by nonoperative management, including physical therapy, image-guided injections, chiropractic care, or behavioral modification including bariatric surgery.

As clinicians, we bring our own biases into the treatment plan for patients and therefore may exhibit heuristic tendencies that drive us toward particular interventions or requests for advanced imaging. A recent study comparing the rate of recommendation for surgery for patients with nonurgent lumbar spine conditions demonstrated that requiring a single visit to a physiatrist decreased surgery rates by 25% [12]. Interestingly, the percentage of fusion procedures within the surgical population increased in this study, suggesting that patients with milder conditions improved with nonoperative management, leaving only the patients with more profound degenerative conditions such as spondylolisthesis or scoliosis to be treated surgically. Studies within the Canadian Health System have demonstrated similar effects [13, 14], noting that patients referred to a dedicated spine pathway that included physiatry experienced less overall MRI utilization while still selecting appropriate surgical candidates for operative intervention. Subsequent analysis from the same group demonstrated that a formalized spine pathway led to improvement in appropriate referrals to spine surgeons, selecting for those patients with the most severe leg pain but without nonspecific back pain who were most likely to benefit from surgery [13, 14]. Even visits with other surgeons seem to reduce the rate of unnecessary surgery, suggesting that this effect isn't solely related to nonsurgeons limiting or denying surgical care options [43, 44]. In both of these studies, a second-opinion surgeon visit led to a recommendation against surgery in 45–50% of patients and a recommendation for a less invasive procedure among many of the remainder.

The use of multidisciplinary team-based approaches is common within cancer care and in some cases is required for accreditation by specialty societies [45]. These venues can serve as a forum to discuss difficult cases but especially in community settings are primarily aimed at helping to standardize care and prevent "outlier" events [46]. This improvement in care is accomplished primarily through a discussion of particular patients by a group of experts from differing fields and capitalizes on what has been called the "wisdom of the crowd" [47]. Both the multidisciplinary spine conference and the multidisciplinary clinic serve the same function as a tumor board: to review the patient's history, examination, and imaging; and to determine a plan of care that has input from the varied specialties involved in the care of this condition. This concept has been utilized routinely throughout many aspects of medical care, but has not yet become a standard of care for the treatment of low back pain, although recent statewide and insurance plan initiatives have proposed the use of such conferences and clinics to help guide patients toward appropriate care [12, 48]. The Robert Bree Collaborative established by the Washington State Legislature, for example, has recently published a lumbar fusion guideline that includes a requirement for "Formal consultation with collaborative team led by board certified physiatrist to confirm appropriateness, adequacy, completeness, and active participation in non-surgical therapy and need for lumbar fusion" as part of its documentation of failure of nonsurgical management [48]. We expect other organizations nationally to follow suit in the face of escalating cost and decreasing value.

Conclusions

Overutilization of spine surgery has led to a decline in the value of care delivered. Rigorous multidisciplinary approaches including multidisciplinary clinics and conferences can decrease the utilization of spine surgery in patients who have questionable benefit from surgical treatment and can thereby provide appropriate care. Ultimately this should improve the value of spine care by removing or reducing the cost of surgery while improving clinical patient outcomes. This, however, is dependent on the availability of coordinated conservative care models. These models of care have been demonstrated to be as effective as spine surgery in conditions such as degenerative axial low back pain and furthermore limit patient's unnecessary exposure to surgical complications when the benefits may be uncertain.

The trend toward value-based spine care represents a tremendous opportunity for providers to take the lead in establishing appropriateness standards to increase the value of spine surgery for patients, purchasers, and health plans alike. While surgeons and medical centers may initially be concerned with lost revenue from cancelled surgeries, better planning can be made when conferences and clinics are held well in advance of a planned surgery. Finally, we feel that the long-term benefits of establishing higher value sustainable spine care will unquestionably be beneficial to all involved. We urge surgeons and nonsurgical clinicians who treat lumbar degenerative conditions to work together to develop the infrastructure necessary to support multidisciplinary approaches to spine care.

References

1. Yanamadala V, Kim Y, Buchlak QD, Wright AK, Babington J, Friedman A, et al. Multidisciplinary evaluation leads to the decreased utilization of lumbar spine fusion. Spine. 2017;42(17):E1016–E23.

2. Castel LD, Freburger JK, Holmes GM, Scheinman RP, Jackman AM, Carey TS. Spine and pain clinics serving North Carolina patients with back and neck pain: what do they do, and are they multidisciplinary? Spine. 2009;34(6):615–22.

3. Vora RN, Barron BA, Almudevar A, Utell MJ. Work-related chronic low back pain-return-to-work outcomes after referral to interventional pain and spine clinics. Spine. 2012;37(20):E1282–9.

4. Barrett PH, Beck A, Schmid K, Fireman B, Brown JB. Treatment decisions about lumbar herniated disk in a shared decision-making program. Jt Comm J Qual Improv. 2002;28(5):211–9.

5. Boss EF, Mehta N, Nagarajan N, Links A, Benke JR, Berger Z, et al. Shared decision making and choice for elective surgical care: a systematic review. Otolaryngol Head Neck Surg. 2016;154(3):405–20.

6. Jones LE, Roberts LC, Little PS, Mullee MA, Cleland JA, Cooper C. Shared decision-making in back pain consultations: an illusion or reality? Eur Spine J. 2014;23(Suppl 1):S13–9.

7. Kim HJ, Park JY, Kang KT, Chang BS, Lee CK, Yeom JS. Factors influencing the surgical decision for the treatment of degenerative lumbar stenosis in a preference-based shared decision-making process. Eur Spine J. 2015;24(2):339–47.

8. Weinstein JN. The missing piece: embracing shared decision making to reform health care. Spine. 2000;25(1):1–4.

9. Kearing S, Berg SZ, Lurie JD. Can decision support help patients with spinal stenosis make a treatment choice? A prospective study assessing the impact of a patient decision aid and health coaching. Spine. 2016;41(7):563–7.

10. Sethi RK, Pong RP, Leveque JC, Dean TC, Olivar SJ, Rupp SM. The Seattle Spine Team approach to adult deformity surgery: a systems-based approach to perioperative care and subsequent reduction in perioperative complication rates. Spine Deform. 2014;2(2):95–103.

11. Halpin RJ, Sugrue PA, Gould RW, Kallas PG, Schafer MF, Ondra SL, et al. Standardizing care for high-risk patients in spine surgery: the Northwestern high-risk spine protocol. Spine. 2010;35(25):2232–8.

12. Fox J, Haig AJ, Todey B, Challa S. The effect of required physiatrist consultation on surgery rates for back pain. Spine. 2013;38(3):E178–84.

13. Kindrachuk DR, Fourney DR. Spine surgery referrals redirected through a multidisciplinary care pathway: effects of nonsurgeon triage including MRI utilization. J Neurosurg Spine. 2014;20(1):87–92.

14. Wilgenbusch CS, Wu AS, Fourney DR. Triage of spine surgery referrals through a multidisciplinary care pathway: a value-based comparison with conventional referral processes. Spine. 2014;39(22 Suppl 1):S129–35.
15. Rasmussen C, Nielsen GL, Hansen VK, Jensen OK, Schioettz-Christensen B. Rates of lumbar disc surgery before and after implementation of multidisciplinary nonsurgical spine clinics. Spine. 2005;30(21):2469–73.
16. Martin BI, Franklin GM, Deyo RA, Wickizer TM, Lurie JD, Mirza SK. How do coverage policies influence practice patterns, safety, and cost of initial lumbar fusion surgery? A population-based comparison of workers' compensation systems. Spine J. 2014;14(7):1237–46.
17. Davis H. Increasing rates of cervical and lumbar spine surgery in the United States, 1979-1990. Spine. 1994;19(10):1117–23; discussion 23-4.
18. Deyo RA, Gray DT, Kreuter W, Mirza S, Martin BI. United States trends in lumbar fusion surgery for degenerative conditions. Spine. 2005;30(12):1441–5; discussion 6-7.
19. Dagostino PR, Whitmore RG, Smith GA, Maltenfort MG, Ratliff JK. Impact of bone morphogenetic proteins on frequency of revision surgery, use of autograft bone, and total hospital charges in surgery for lumbar degenerative disease: review of the Nationwide inpatient sample from 2002 to 2008. Spine J. 2014;14(1):20–30.
20. Weinstein JN, Lurie JD, Olson PR, Bronner KK, Fisher ES. United States' trends and regional variations in lumbar spine surgery: 1992-2003. Spine. 2006;31(23):2707–14.
21. Thirukumaran CP, Raudenbush B, Li Y, Molinari R, Rubery P, Mesfin A. National trends in the surgical management of adult lumbar isthmic spondylolisthesis: 1998 to 2011. Spine. 2016;41(6):490–501.
22. Yoshihara H, Yoneoka D. National trends in the surgical treatment for lumbar degenerative disc disease: United States, 2000 to 2009. Spine J. 2015;15(2):265–71.
23. Lad SP, Patil CG, Berta S, Santarelli JG, Ho C, Boakye M. National trends in spinal fusion for cervical spondylotic myelopathy. Surg Neurol. 2009;71(1):66–9; discussion 9.
24. Rajaee SS, Bae HW, Kanim LE, Delamarter RB. Spinal fusion in the United States: analysis of trends from 1998 to 2008. Spine. 2012;37(1):67–76.
25. Mehrotra C, Remington PL, Naimi TS, Washington W, Miller R. Trends in total knee replacement surgeries and implications for public health, 1990-2000. Public Health Rep. 2005;120(3):278–82.
26. Lysaght MJ. Maintenance dialysis population dynamics: current trends and long-term implications. J Am Soc Nephrol. 2002;13(Suppl 1):S37–40.
27. Neumann PJ, Cohen JT, Weinstein MC. Updating cost-effectiveness--the curious resilience of the $50,000-per-QALY threshold. N Engl J Med. 2014;371(9):796–7.

28. Chang RW, Pellisier JM, Hazen GB. A cost-effectiveness analysis of total hip arthroplasty for osteoarthritis of the hip. JAMA. 1996;275(11):858–65.
29. Carreon LY, Anderson PA, Traynelis VC, Mummaneni PV, Glassman SD. Cost-effectiveness of single-level anterior cervical discectomy and fusion five years after surgery. Spine. 2013;38(6):471–5.
30. Meyer SA, Mummaneni PV. Cost-effectiveness of transforaminal lumbar interbody fusion. J Neurosurg Spine. 2011;15(2):136–7; discussion 7.
31. Mummaneni PV, Whitmore RG, Curran JN, Ziewacz JE, Wadhwa R, Shaffrey CI, et al. Cost-effectiveness of lumbar discectomy and single-level fusion for spondylolisthesis: experience with the NeuroPoint-SD registry. Neurosurg Focus. 2014;36(6):E3.
32. Hedlund R, Johansson C, Hagg O, Fritzell P, Tullberg T. Swedish Lumbar Spine Study G. The long-term outcome of lumbar fusion in the Swedish lumbar spine study. Spine J. 2016;16(5):579–87.
33. Nguyen TH, Randolph DC, Talmage J, Succop P, Travis R. Long-term outcomes of lumbar fusion among workers' compensation subjects: a historical cohort study. Spine. 2011;36(4):320–31.
34. Lingutla KK, Pollock R, Benomran E, Purushothaman B, Kasis A, Bhatia CK, et al. Outcome of lumbar spinal fusion surgery in obese patients: a systematic review and meta-analysis. Bone Joint J. 2015;97-B(10):1395–404.
35. Asghar FA, Hilibrand AS. The impact of the Spine Patient Outcomes Research Trial (SPORT) results on orthopaedic practice. J Am Acad Orthop Surg. 2012;20(3):160–6.
36. Birkmeyer NJ, Weinstein JN, Tosteson AN, Tosteson TD, Skinner JS, Lurie JD, et al. Design of the Spine Patient outcomes Research Trial (SPORT). Spine. 2002;27(12):1361–72.
37. Hart RA, The Spine Patient Outcomes Research Trial (SPORT): a continuing return on investment: commentary on an article by Jeffrey A. Rihn, MD, et al. The influence of obesity on the outcome of treatment of lumbar disc herniation. Analysis of the Spine Patient Outcomes Research Trial (SPORT). J Bone Joint Surg Am. 2013;95(1):e5.
38. Levin PE. The impact of the Spine Patient Outcome Research Trial (SPORT) results on orthopaedic practice. J Am Acad Orthop Surg. 2012;20(6):331; author reply -2.
39. Lurie JD, Tosteson TD, Tosteson A, Abdu WA, Zhao W, Morgan TS, et al. Long-term outcomes of lumbar spinal stenosis: eight-year results of the Spine Patient Outcomes Research Trial (SPORT). Spine. 2015;40(2):63–76.
40. Directors NASSBo. Spine Patient Outcome Research Trial (SPORT): multi-center randomized clinical trial of surgical and non-surgical approaches to the treatment of low back pain. Spine J. 2003;3(6):417–9.
41. Park DK, An HS, Lurie JD, Zhao W, Tosteson A, Tosteson TD, et al. Does multilevel lumbar stenosis lead to poorer outcomes? A subanalysis of the Spine Patient Outcomes Research Trial (SPORT) lumbar stenosis study. Spine. 2010;35(4):439–46.

42. Weinstein JN, Tosteson AN, Tosteson TD, Lurie JD, Abdu WA, Mirza SK, et al. The SPORT value compass: do the extra costs of undergoing spine surgery produce better health benefits? Med Care. 2014;52(12):1055–63.

43. Gamache FW. The value of "another" opinion for spinal surgery: a prospective 14-month study of one surgeon's experience. Surg Neurol Int. 2012;3(Suppl 5):S350–4.

44. Vialle E. Second opinion in spine surgery: a Brazilian perspective. Eur J Orthop Surg Traumatol. 2015;25(Suppl 1):S3–6.

45. Winchester DP. The United States' national accreditation program for breast centers: a model for excellence in breast disease evaluation and management. Chin Clin Oncol. 2016;5(3):31.

46. Gross GE. The role of the tumor board in a community hospital. CA Cancer J Clin. 1987;37(2):88–92.

47. Surowiecki J. The wisdom of crowds: why the many are smarter than the few and how collective wisdom shapes business, economies, societies, and nations. 1st ed. New York: Doubleday; 2004. xxi, 296 p.

48. Available from: http://www.breecollaborative.org/.

Using Lean Process Improvement to Enhance Safety and Value

5

Michael A. Bohl and Gary S. Kaplan

What Is Standard Work?

Following the Allied victory in World War II, Japanese industrialists began studying the American manufacturing processes that enabled the USA to achieve previously unheard of productivity and efficiency in manufacturing (some US plants boasted they were building "a bomber an hour" during the height of the war). The founders of Toyota, for example, combined certain aspects of the Ford system with their own theories on continual process improvement, minimization of waste, and work standardization. The result was the development of the Toyota Production System (TPS) and many of the founding principles of what we refer to today as "lean methodology." With these principles in practice, Japanese manufacturing was revolutionized into a dominant industrial force of the twentieth century [1, 2].

M. A. Bohl
Department of Neurosurgery, Barrow Neurological Institute,
St. Joseph's Hospital and Medical Center, Phoenix, AZ, USA

G. S. Kaplan (✉)
Virginia Mason Medical Center, Seattle, WA, USA
e-mail: Gary.Kaplan@virginiamason.org

© Springer Nature Switzerland AG 2020
R. K. Sethi et al. (eds.), *Value-Based Approaches to Spine Care*,
https://doi.org/10.1007/978-3-030-31946-5_5

The TPS comprises a management philosophy centered on core principles of waste minimization and iterative improvements in work processes. A central tenet of the TPS is the development of standard work processes. The concept of standard work was developed by Japanese engineer Taiichi Ohno as a means of achieving incremental improvement (*kaizen*) in any work process. The concept of *kaizen* is best summarized by Taiichi Ohno himself, who said, "Without standards, there can be no improvement." In other words, when work is non-standardized, unpredictable, and highly variable over time, it is impossible to know which components of a work process are adding value and which are adding waste. By establishing a consistent work process with known outcomes (the "standard" work), one creates what is effectively a control group against which future iterative changes to the work process can be compared. Any changes that result in better outcomes are adopted as part of the new standard work process, and any changes that result in worse outcomes are discarded from the process as waste. Improvement in a work process can therefore only be made after establishing a standard work process and identifying the correct process and quality metrics (the outcomes) to measure [2–7].

To standardize a work process, that process must first be deconstructed into discrete steps, and each step detailed according to (1) the person conducting the work, (2) the task itself, and (3) the check process to ensure the work was done sufficiently. By deconstructing work in this fashion, one is able to both establish standards for work performance and identify problems in the work process that prevent achievement of the standard. After a standard is established, incremental improvements in each step of the work process are made in order to improve the entire process. The people responsible for carrying out a work process are furthermore empowered to identify waste in the process or areas of potential improvement and therefore become an essential part of the iterative improvement process [2, 5–7].

The Toyota Production System and Its Application in Healthcare

The success of the TPS in automotive manufacturing has inspired its use in other industries such as diverse manufacturing industries, food service, air travel, retail, and healthcare. Although modifications to the TPS methodology are required when applied to human services industries, the core principles of standard work, continual process improvement, and personnel empowerment remain unchanged. Companies such as Southwest Airlines, Walmart, and Taco Bell have made tremendous gains in productivity and customer satisfaction after employing lean methodologies. These gains have inspired many in healthcare to adopt these same methods [8–20].

In 2002, the Virginia Mason Medical Center became one of the first healthcare institutions to employ lean methods in a hospital-wide attempt to improve the quality of delivered patient care [2]. The impact at Virginia Mason on certain standard quality metrics was astounding: within 2 years of implementing lean methodologies, incidences of ventilator-associated pneumonia at Virginia Mason decreased from 34 cases and 5 deaths annually to 4 cases and 1 death. Annual cost saving to the hospital from this reduction alone was reported to be $500,000 [2, 20–23]. Around the same time, large hospital systems in Pennsylvania and Wisconsin began employing lean methodologies with similarly substantive improvements reported over the following years. The Pittsburgh Regional Health Initiative, for example, achieved a 90% reduction in central line infections within the first year of implementing lean methods to their quality control efforts. ThedaCare in Wisconsin reported $3.3 million in overall institutional savings after implementing their own lean program targeted at identifying and eliminating waste [24].

These early successes in implementing lean methodologies in healthcare settings inspired widespread adoption of lean practices over the past decade throughout nearly every type of healthcare facility and practice setting, from trauma to ambulatory care centers, from academic to private hospital systems, and in fields from family medicine to subspecialty surgery. In some of these examples, successful implementation of TPS principles relied heavily on an institution-wide adoption of certain cultural changes, including empowerment of individuals and a willingness and commitment to make iterative changes in order to achieve continuous process improvement.

What Is the Virginia Mason Production System? How Does This System Root Out Variability?

The early success of lean methodologies applied in the Virginia Mason Medical Center inspired the development of the Virginia Mason Production System (VMPS), an adaptation of the TPS on a medical center-wide scale [21]. A keystone principle of the VMPS is the establishment of a healthcare culture in which each person is empowered to examine work processes and implement changes in those processes to achieve continuous improvement. Hospital leadership is responsible for creating and supporting this culture from the top down, as well as providing comprehensive oversight of ongoing work processes, instituted changes, and the results of these changes on process outcomes. By their nature, lean processes are continually evolving; the VMPS has created its own system for systematically monitoring the changes that have been implemented and the effect of these changes on work processes over time. After having been in place for over a decade, the VMPS has achieved annual systematic reductions in cost and medical errors throughout the Virginia Mason Medical Center. As a result, the VMPS principles have been extended into certain high-risk, high-cost specialties such as orthopedic surgery and neurosurgery [22–35].

The ability of the VMPS to achieve continuous improvement in healthcare outcomes is dependent on its ability to root out variability in healthcare work processes. After targeting a value-focused area of potential improvement, the first step in the VMPS is to deconstruct the work processes involved and to define those processes in terms of the task, the person conducting the task, and monitoring of task performance. Once this is accomplished, a task performance standard can be established, and all persons performing that task can be evaluated in respect to the new standard. Variables in task performance that result in above or below standard outcomes can then be identified, changes to the work processes that favor above standard work can be iteratively implemented, and over time the variability in work process performance is eliminated in favor of best practices.

Cultural Aspects of Hierarchy in Medicine and Surgery (the Old Standard Way)

The application of an automotive manufacturing management philosophy to a field as complex as healthcare is fraught with challenges. First, healthcare does not function like most business entities in which there is a single hierarchy of decision-making authority and a single CEO ultimately responsible for the collective success or failure of the company. In healthcare, every physician involved in the care of a patient has traditionally functioned essentially as their own CEO, ultimately responsible for the success or failure of their own patient management decisions, while each patient's eventual outcome is often dependent on the collective impact of multiple physicians' and team member's input. The notion of standardizing work processes in a system with such diffuse decision-making authority and disparate work processes is daunting. Furthermore, many physicians are wary of systems in which their own decision-making process can be supplanted or changed, as they will ultimately be responsible (and legally liable) for their patients' outcomes and satisfaction. This is evolving in recent years with the enhanced understanding of the role of teams and physicians as team leaders and team members.

Secondly, the type of work conducted across different healthcare settings varies significantly from easily defined processes (i.e., patient transportation, bed turnover, blood draws) to much more ambiguous processes such as medical decision-making. When applied to unambiguous and easily articulated tasks such as central venous line or endotracheal tube management protocols, lean process method-ologies can readily be employed [8–19]. But when applied to more complex tasks that require rapid decision-making based on numerous information streams from sources of variable reliability, the notion of task deconstruction and standardization becomes more difficult. These complex types of work processes can more broadly be defined as "knowledge work." Knowledge work requires an expert in a given area (i.e., a physician) to collect information from various sources and then synthesize that information to make a decision. The mental work processes that dictate the physician's decision-making process are often ambiguous and unpredictable and rely heavily on physi-cian experience and tacit knowledge, the "art" of medicine. Some believe that because knowledge work is not repetitive and cannot be unambiguously defined, this type of work is not well-suited for lean methodologies [42].

The impact of these challenges on healthcare quality improve-ment has been a split in the type of work processes that generally undergo lean process development. Hospital tasks that are largely overseen by nursing and nonphysician staff have a long-track record of success in improving quality metrics after lean practices are implemented. Physicians, on the other hand, have been more skeptical and slower to adopt lean practices as their work processes are more difficult to standardize, and the hierarchy of decision-making authority in which they operate is highly fractionated. Thus, the old standard way of practice continues to prevail at many institutions, individual physicians performing the same tasks using widely disparate work processes and achieving highly variable results. When work is non-standardized, unpredictable, or highly variable in this fashion, it is impossible to establish a standard and therefore difficult to nearly impossible to know how to improve the work and demonstrate enhancements in quality.

Adult Spinal Deformity Surgery as a Case Study (the Need for Change)

The shortcomings of the old, non-standardized way of delivering healthcare are most readily seen in the performance of our highest-risk surgical procedures. Surgical corrections of adult spinal deformities, for example, are among the most dangerous operations in the surgical armamentarium, with reported morbidity rates ranging from 20% to nearly 90% [43–45]. Intraoperative adverse events are reportedly as high as 10% in these procedures and include temporary or permanent neurological deficit, high-volume blood loss, myocardial infarction, stroke, and/or death [22–29]. There are several reports in the literature of patients who lost more than their total preoperative estimated blood volume during a corrective spinal fusion for scoliosis. As the incidence of degenerative spinal deformity has grown with our aging population and the demand for surgical corrections of these deformities has likewise grown, the same phenomenon has continued through the current decade [46–54]. But despite the morbidity of these procedures, many patients report significant improvements in their quality of life following reconstruction of their spinal deformities, even those who suffer the aforementioned complications [55–67]. The onus is therefore on surgeons to develop strategies for minimizing risk for patients in whom surgery is the only feasible treatment option.

Given the high morbidity and mortality of adult scoliosis correction procedures, there is a growing need to develop strategies aimed at reducing the risk of these procedures. The delivery of surgical care to patients with complex spinal deformities requires a large number of steps across complex healthcare systems that must be completed to take a patient from the beginning to the end of the "production line." These steps broadly include preoperative work, intraoperative work, and postoperative work. Given individual surgeon variability in training, expertise, and personal experience, the amount of variability and potential for error in the overall work processes surrounding complex surgical spine care is staggering. As such, the delivery of surgical treatment for complex spine deformities lends itself very well to standardized work processes.

Lean methodologies offer a number of potential benefits to spinal reconstructive procedures as many aspects of these procedures lend themselves well to work process deconstruction and standardization. For example, some centers have developed custom protocols designed to minimize individual complications, such as blood loss or postoperative vision loss [36–39]. Others have found success implementing even broader lean protocols, with improvements in outcomes and reduced overall complication rates [40, 41].

The Seattle Spine Team Approach
(the New Standard Way)

Prior to the application of broad lean process improvement strategies and standard work principles to the care of adult spinal deformity patients at Virginia Mason, the work processes in place around the care of these patients were highly variable and of unpredictable quality. Complication rates for these procedures were over 50% [40]. After the occurrence of two major complications (a debilitating stroke and intraoperative death), the surgical treatment of all spinal deformities was halted. In car manufacturing, the TPS calls for a production line to be stopped when someone identifies a situation leading to production of a poor-quality vehicle. This same "stop the line" strategy was implemented at Virginia Mason after it became clear that the "production line" for surgical reconstruction of spinal deformities was producing bad outcomes. With the production line stopped, physician stakeholders and hospital personnel were able to conduct root cause analyses to identify numerous areas for potential systems improvement. The end result was a radical reconstruction of the entire work process, an event known in TPS terminology as *kaikaku*.

The Seattle Spine Team Approach (SSTA) was the standard work process that resulted from this kaikaku approach and is just one example of the broad and systematic application of lean principles to the performance of adult reconstructive spine surgery. Most importantly, the SSTA represents a case study in how lean methodologies can successfully be applied to complex surgical procedures. The first challenge in implementing the SSTA was to define value in scoliosis correction procedures. Although this step may seem intuitive, it is imperative that all key service providers involved in these procedures (surgeons, anesthesiologists, physiatrists, internists, pain specialists, nurses, operating room staff, physician assistants) are included so as to bring together a multidisciplinary perspective on the numerous work processes involved and which outcomes are most important to measure. By including all stakeholders, one furthermore empowers those performing the various tasks required during these procedures to implement change; staff empowerment is one of the key principles of lean manufacturing. Key service providers identified by the SSTA team worked together in a rapid process improvement workshop and collectively defined value as delivering the safest and most effective complex spine surgery at the lowest cost [68].

The next step was to deconstruct the various work processes involved in a complex surgical spine procedure into a standardized work process. To do this, a value stream map was created that incorporates preoperative, perioperative, and postoperative care into a single process flow map. This map delineates each of the steps involved in delivering the defined value (safe, effective surgery at the lowest cost). As this process of value streaming is iteratively performed, current state maps are generated in which each area of the work process for conducting a surgical spine correction is studied in detail to identify waste in the process. Each step in the process can be detailed as broadly or specifically as necessary, depending on the focus of a particular improvement effort. Areas that do not immediately relate to the focus of an improvement effort can be depicted very broadly, whereas those that are directly related are detailed very specifically. This granular view of a particular part of the work process then enables further deconstruction of that task in terms of standardized work: who is performing the task, what is the task, and how is task performance evaluated. Areas of potential improvement are thus identified, and the implementation of changes to the process is initiated [68].

It is important to maintain direct communication with the personnel involved in each process that is identified as a focus area of improvement. In the SSTA, the people involved in the identified tasks are interviewed in the setting of a process improvement workshop focused on identifying waste and inefficiencies in the existing work process. After an intervention is agreed upon, a future state map is created to analyze the ideal value stream that is expected to result from the intervention. This future state value stream is similarly deconstructed into its component standard work to ensure the new value stream is performed as intended and that the intended improvements are made and maintained over time [68].

The desired intervention is then implemented in real time by personnel responsible for the new work process. Assessment of outcome parameters begins immediately and is conducted continuously so that managers can monitor the level of improvement over time. Once the future state value stream is achieved, this value stream becomes the new standard against which all future value streams are compared. This process is then repeated in an iterative process of continuous self-evaluation and improvement [68].

After the SSTA was implemented in this fashion, the overall complication rate for complex spine surgery was reduced from 52% to 16%, and this improvement has been sustained for over 5 years of continuous lean process improvement in preoperative screening, intraoperative communication strategies, complication avoidance protocols, and postoperative care pathways [40]. This continuous process of self-evaluation and iterative changes to work processes is felt by the SSTA team to be essential to maintaining and building on this improvement over time.

Potential Pitfalls and Areas for Improvement

Collective Intelligence or Groupthink?

Minimization of work process variability is a critical principle in the formation of a standard work process like the SSTA. One of the greatest challenges in standardizing this sort of comprehensive work process is to root out variability in the knowledge work phases of the production line. These phases of work typically require knowledge experts (physicians, in this case) to synthesize information from numerous sources of variable reliability in order to come up with a single best treatment plan. Numerous studies have shown that when presented the same information streams (e.g., patient histories, laboratory values, medical imaging studies, etc.), different experts not only produce very different treatment strategies from each other, but will also produce different treatment strategies from themselves when presented the same case after allowing for a period of time to pass [69, 70]. To minimize this variability in knowledge work phases of production, the

SSTA implements a multidisciplinary, shared decision-making conference comprised of experts from all stakeholder specialties in the care of spinal deformity patients. All members of this conference have equal authority and input to the decision-making process, and a consensus must be reached by the conference before a final treatment plan is agreed on. This system is meant to minimize variability by distributing decision-making input and authority to numerous expert providers, reasoning that in complex decision-making, more heads are better than one.

Some debate exists, however, around the utility of shared decision-making among a group of experts. Proponents of multidisciplinary conferences cite a growing body of literature on the ability of groups of experts to outperform single individuals in complex decision-making tasks [71–76]. This concept is known as collective intelligence or the "wisdom of crowds" and has been demonstrated to exist across a number of species, from microbes to humans [77–80]. For example, groups of radiologists have been shown to outperform the single most accurate radiologist in the interpretation of mammograms [74, 75]. Some argue, however, that multidisciplinary committees are prone to a harmful psychological phenomenon known as "groupthink," in which a desire for harmony and group conformity leads to irrational or dysfunctional decision-making through the suppression of dissenting viewpoints, especially when those viewpoints contradict group leaders [71–73, 81]. It is therefore important for groups that have implemented these conferences to monitor conference outcomes and perform objective, in-depth analyses of how the conference functions, how decisions are made, and what impact the conference is having on patient care and surgical decision-making. For example, anonymous voting data on physician opinions about specific cases of degenerative spine disease have been collected over time as part of the SSTA's continuous process improvement efforts. This data suggests that treatment biases exist among both individual surgeon and non-surgeon members of the conference and surgeons and non-surgeons as groups of physicians. It is important to identify these biases as they may introduce more variability into the decision-making process depending on which members of the conference participate and how much input they provide.

A paucity of published data exists on this topic as it applies to spinal deformities. The notion of collective intelligence, however, has been widely described and studied in other fields, and future efforts to apply collective intelligence to the field of complex spine surgery should focus on the specific model of collective intelligence used. Numerous models of collective intelligence have been described, each with variable accuracies and data requirements for implementation. For example, collective intelligence systems generally operate via one of four different decision-making models: confidence-based models (the most confident group member makes the decision), simple majority models (the most popular vote wins), quorum-based models (a decision-making threshold is established based on a known group accuracy), and weighted-quorum models (individual voters have weighted input based on their known individual accuracies). Group accuracy increases as one moves from the confidence-based model to the weighted-quorum model [74]. Future studies on the effects of multidisciplinary conferences as applied to complex surgical spine care should evaluate conference outcomes in this framework and with this level of granularity. Future studies should also evaluate patient perceptions of collective intelligence decision-making systems in their own care. In our own experience, patients often express appreciation for the team approach to diagnosis and treatment recommendations. It should also be noted that patients express appreciation for the "team" approach to evaluation and recommended intervention.

Patient Optimization or Restriction of Care?

Significant debate currently exists around the true impact of multidisciplinary, shared decision-making conferences. Proponents of multidisciplinary conferences argue that a preoperative evaluation and strict surgical clearance process results in better optimization of patients with subsequent improved outcomes and cost savings to the health system. Critics of these conferences argue the improved outcomes are simply a result of restricting care to a healthier subset of patients who would predictably have better outcomes following any surgical procedure. The intention of the SSTA is not to restrict care to a smaller subset of healthier patients but to provide better preoperative optimization for all patients with subsequent delivery of surgical care to all those who stand to benefit. Although no published data exists yet on this topic, early results from the SSTA's own internal review of complex spine conference outcomes suggest the possibility that the current multidisciplinary conference is currently removing a large percentage of patients from the surgical population and that these patients comprise a higher-risk subset of patients. If, in fact, these conferences are achieving improved results due at least in part to restriction of care, institutions employing these conferences will need to devise new strategies to ensure that patients who stand to gain the most from surgery, even if they pose a higher surgical risk, are not being marginalized for the sake of better institutional statistics. It is important to remember in the application of lean manufacturing principles to healthcare settings that success should not be defined by institutional financial success, but by the improvement in patient quality of life being delivered.

References

1. Call R. 'Lean' approach gives greater efficiency. Health Estate. 2014;68(2):23–5.
2. Kim CS, Spahlinger DA, Kin JM, Billi JE. Lean health care: what can hospitals learn from a world-class automaker? J Hosp Med. 2006;1(3):191–9.
3. Spear SJ. Learning to lead at Toyota. Harv Bus Rev. 2004;82(5):78–86, 151.
4. Clark DM, Silvester K, Knowles S. Lean management systems: creating a culture of continuous quality improvement. J Clin Pathol. 2013;66(8):638–43.
5. Womack JP, Jones DT. Lean consumption. Harv Bus Rev. 2005;83(3):58–68, 148.
6. Girdler SJ, Glezos CD, Link TM, Sharan A. The science of quality improvement. JBJS Rev. 2016;4(8):1.
7. Weinstock D. Lean healthcare. J Med Pract Manage. 2008;23(6):339–41.
8. Jimmerson C, Weber D, Sobek DK II. Reducing waste and errors: piloting lean principles at Intermountain Healthcare. Jt Comm J Qual Patient Saf. 2005;31(5):249–57.
9. Kinsman L, Rotter T, Stevenson K, et al. "The largest lean transformation in the world": the implementation and evaluation of lean in Saskatchewan healthcare. Healthc Q. 2014;17(2):29–32.

10. Blayney DW. Measuring and improving quality of care in an academic medical center. J Oncol Pract. 2013;9(3):138–41.
11. Pittsburgh Regional Healthcare Initiative puts new spin on improving healthcare quality. Qual Lett Healthc Lead. 2002;14(11):2–11, 1.
12. Brown T, Duthe R. Getting 'lean': hardwiring process excellence into Northeast Health. J Healthc Inf Manag. 2009;23(1):34–8.
13. Casey JT, Brinton TS, Gonzalez CM. Utilization of lean management principles in the ambulatory clinic setting. Nat Clin Pract Urol. 2009;6(3):146–53.
14. Serembus JF, Meloy F, Posmontier B. Learning from business: incorporating the Toyota production system into nursing curricula. Nurs Clin North Am. 2012;47(4):503–16.
15. Rutledge J, Xu M, Simpson J. Application of the Toyota production system improves core laboratory operations. Am J Clin Pathol. 2010;133(1):24–31.
16. Serrano L, Hegge P, Sato B, Richmond B, Stahnke L. Using LEAN principles to improve quality, patient safety, and workflow in histology and anatomic pathology. Adv Anat Pathol. 2010;17(3):215–21.
17. Stapleton FB, Hendricks J, Hagan P, DelBeccaro M. Modifying the Toyota production system for continuous performance improvement in an academic children's hospital. Pediatr Clin N Am. 2009;56(4):799–813.
18. Teichgräber UK, de Bucourt M. Applying value stream mapping techniques to eliminate non-value-added waste for the procurement of endovascular stents. Eur J Radiol. 2012;81(1):e47–52.
19. Burkitt KH, Mor MK, Jain R, et al. Toyota production system quality improvement initiative improves perioperative antibiotic therapy. Am J Manag Care. 2009;15(9):633–42.
20. Bradywood A, Farrokhi F, Williams B, Kowalczyk M, Blackmore CC. Reduction of inpatient hospital length of stay in lumbar fusion patients with implementation of an evidence-based clinical care pathway. Spine (Phila Pa 1976). 2017;42(3):169–76.
21. Nelson-Peterson DL, Leppa CJ. Creating an environment for caring using lean principles of the Virginia Mason production system. J Nurs Adm. 2007;37(6):287–94.
22. Rampersaud YR, Moro ER, Neary MA, et al. Intraoperative adverse events and related postoperative complications in spine surgery: implications for enhancing patient safety founded on evidence-based protocols. Spine (Phila Pa 1976). 2006;31(13):1503–10.
23. Bertram W, Harding I. Complications of spinal deformity and spinal stenosis surgery in adults greater than 50 years old. Orthop Proc. 2012;94(suppl X):105.
24. Booth KC, Bridwell KH, Lenke LG, Baldus CR, Blanke KM. Complications and predictive factors for the successful treatment of flatback deformity (fixed sagittal imbalance). Spine (Phila Pa 1976). 1999;24(16):1712–20.

25. Cho SK, Bridwell KH, Lenke LG, et al. Major complications in revision adult deformity surgery: risk factors and clinical outcomes with 2- to 7-year follow-up. Spine (Phila Pa 1976). 2012;37(6):489–500.
26. Daubs MD, Lenke LG, Cheh G, Stobbs G, Bridwell KH. Adult spinal deformity surgery: complications and outcomes in patients over age 60. Spine (Phila Pa 1976). 2007;32(20):2238–44.
27. Glassman SD, Hamill CL, Bridwell KH, Schwab FJ, Dimar JR, Lowe TG. The impact of perioperative complications on clinical outcome in adult deformity surgery. Spine (Phila Pa 1976). 2007;32(24):2764–70.
28. Schwab FJ, Hawkinson N, Lafage V, Smith JS, Hart R, Mundis G, Burton DC, Line B, Akbarnia B, Boachie-Adjei O, Hostin R, International Spine Study Group. Risk factors for major peri-operative complications in adult spinal deformity surgery: a multi-center review of 953 consecutive patients. Eur Spine J. 2012;21(12):2603–10.
29. Lenke LG, Fehlings MG, Shaffrey CI, Cheung KM, Carreon LY. Prospective, multicenter assessment of acute neurologic complications following complex adult spinal deformity surgery: the Scoli-Risk-1 trial. Spine J. 2013;13(9 suppl):S67.
30. Acosta FL Jr, McClendon J Jr, O'Shaughnessy BA, et al. Morbidity and mortality after spinal deformity surgery in patients 75 years and older: complications and predictive factors. J Neurosurg Spine. 2011;15(6):667–74.
31. Kaplan GS, Patterson SH. Seeking perfection in healthcare: a case study in adopting Toyota production system methods. Healthc Exec. 2008;23(3):16–8, 20–21.
32. Yanamadala V, Kim Y, Buchlak QD, et al. Multidisciplinary evaluation leads to the decreased utilization of lumbar spine fusion: an observational cohort pilot study. Spine (Phila Pa 1976). 2017;42:E1016–23.
33. Institute for Healthcare Improvement: Innovation series 2005. Going lean in healthcare. https://www.entnet.org/sites/default/files/GoingLeanin HealthCareWhitePaper-3.pdf. Accessed 31 Aug 2017.
34. Buchlak QD, Yanamadala V, Leveque JC, Sethi R. Complication avoidance with pre-operative screening: insights from the Seattle spine team. Curr Rev Musculoskelet Med. 2016;9(3):316–26.
35. Allen RT, Rihn JA, Glassman SD, Currier B, Albert TJ, Phillips FM. An evidence- based approach to spine surgery. Am J Med Qual. 2009;24(6 suppl):15S–24S.
36. Ames CP, Barry JJ, Keshavarzi S, Dede O, Weber MH, Deviren V. Perioperative outcomes and complications of pedicle subtraction osteotomy in cases with single versus two attending surgeons. Spine Deform. 2013;1(1):51–8.
37. Baig MN, Lubow M, Immesoete P, Bergese SD, Hamdy EA, Mendel E. Vision loss after spine surgery: review of the literature and recommendations. Neurosurg Focus. 2007;23(5):E15.
38. Baldus CR, Bridwell KH, Lenke LG, Okubadejo GO. Can we safely reduce blood loss during lumbar pedicle subtraction osteotomy procedures

using tranexamic acid or aprotinin? A comparative study with controls. Spine (Phila Pa 1976). 2010;35(2):235–9.

39. Urban MK, Beckman J, Gordon M, Urquhart B, Boachie-Adjei O. The efficacy of antifibrinolytics in the reduction of blood loss during complex adult reconstructive spine surgery. Spine (Phila Pa 1976). 2001;26(10):1152–6.

40. Sethi RK, Pong RP, Leveque JC, Dean TC, Olivar SJ, Rupp SM. The Seattle spine team approach to adult deformity surgery: a systems-based approach to perioperative care and subsequent reduction in perioperative complication rates. Spine Deform. 2014;2(2):95–103.

41. Sethi R, Buchlak QD, Yanamadala V, et al. A systematic multidisciplinary initiative for reducing the risk of complications in adult scoliosis surgery. J Neurosurg Spine. 2017;26(6):744–50.

42. Staats B, Upton D. Lean knowledge work. Harv Bus Rev. 2011. Accessed online https://hbr.org/2011/10/lean-knowledge-work. 2-20-2019.

43. Howe CR, Agel J, Lee MJ, et al. The morbidity and mortality of fusions from the thoracic spine to the pelvis in the adult population. Spine (Phila Pa 1976). 2011;36:1397–401.

44. Schwab FJ, Hawkinson N, Lafage V, et al. Risk factors for major perioperative complications in adult spinal deformity surgery: a multi-center review of 953 consecutive patients. Eur Spine J. 2012;21:2603e10.

45. Street JT, Lenehan BJ, DiPaola CP, et al. Morbidity and mortality of major adult spinal surgery. A prospective cohort analysis of 942 consecutive patients. Spine J. 2012;12:22–34.

46. Tormenti MJ, et al. Perioperative surgical complications of transforaminal lumbar interbody fusion: a single-center experience. J Neurosurg Spine. 2012;16(1):44–50.

47. Guay J, Haig M, Lortie L, et al. Predicting blood loss in surgery for idiopathic scoliosis. Can J Anaesth. 1994;41:775e81.

48. Guay J, Reinberg C, Poitras B, et al. A trial of desmopressin to reduce blood loss in patients undergoing spinal fusion for idiopathic scoliosis. Anesth Analg. 1992;75:405e10.

49. Phillips WA, Hensinger RN. Control of blood loss during scoliosis surgery. Clin Orthop Rel Res. 1988;229:88e93.

50. Uden A, Nilsson IM, Willner S. Collagen-induced platelet aggregation and bleeding time in adolescent idiopathic scoliosis. Acta Orthop Scand. 1980;51:773e7.

51. Egafy H, Bransford RJ, McGuire RA, et al. Blood loss in major spine surgery: are there effective measures to decrease massive hemorrhage in major spine fusion surgery? Spine (Phila Pa 1976). 2010;35(9 Suppl):S47e56.

52. Modi HN, Suh SW, Hong JY, et al. Intraoperative blood loss during different stages of scoliosis surgery: a prospective study. Scoliosis. 2010;5:16.

53. Baldus CR, Bridwell KH, Lenke LG, et al. Can we safely reduce blood loss during lumbar pedicle subtraction osteotomy procedures using

tranexamic acid or aprotinin? A comparative study with controls. Spine (Phila Pa 1976). 2010;35:235e9.

54. Yu X, Xiao H, Wang R, et al. Prediction of massive blood loss in scoliosis surgery from preoperative variables. Spine (Phila Pa 1976). 2013;38:350e5.

55. Bridwell KH, Baldus C, Berven S, et al. Changes in radiographic and clinical outcomes with primary treatment adult spinal deformity surgeries from two years to three- to five-years follow-up. Spine (Phila Pa 1976). 2010;35:1849–54.

56. Bridwell KH, Glassman S, Horton W, et al. Does treatment (nonoperative and operative) improve the two-year quality of life in patients with adult symptomatic lumbar scoliosis: a prospective multicenter evidence-based medicine study. Spine (Phila Pa 1976). 2009;34:2171–8.

57. Liu S, Schwab F, Smith JS, et al. Likelihood of reaching minimal clinically important difference in adult spinal deformity: a comparison of operative and nonoperative treatment. Ochsner J. 2014;14:67–77.

58. Scheer JK, Smith JS, Clark AJ, et al. Comprehensive study of back and leg pain improvements after adult spinal deformity surgery: analysis of 421 patients with 2-year follow-up and of the impact of the surgery on treatment satisfaction. J Neurosurg Spine. 2015;22:540–53.

59. Smith JS, Kasliwal MK, Crawford A, et al. Outcomes, expectations, and complications overview for the surgical treatment of adult and pediatric spinal deformity. Spine Deform. 2012;(Preview Issue):4–14.

60. Smith JS, Klineberg E, Schwab F, et al. Change in classification grade by the SRS-Schwab Adult Spinal Deformity Classification predicts impact on health-related quality of life measures: prospective analysis of operative and nonoperative treatment. Spine (Phila Pa 1976). 2013;38:1663–71.

61. Smith JS, Lafage V, Shaffrey CI, et al. Outcomes of operative and nonoperative treatment for adult spinal deformity: a prospective, multi-center matched cohort assessment with 2-year follow-up. Neurosurgery. 2016;78:851–61.

62. Smith JS, Shaffrey CI, Berven S, et al. Operative versus nonoperative treatment of leg pain in adults with scoliosis: a retrospective review of a prospective multicenter database with two-year follow-up. Spine (Phila Pa 1976). 2009;34:1693–8.

63. Smith JS, Shaffrey CI, Berven S, et al. Improvement of back pain with operative and nonoperative treatment in adults with scoliosis. Neurosurgery. 2009;65:86–93.

64. Smith JS, Shaffrey CI, Glassman SD, et al. Risk-benefit assessment of surgery for adult scoliosis: an analysis based on patient age. Spine (Phila Pa 1976). 2011;36:817–24.

65. Smith JS, Shaffrey CI, Glassman SD, et al. Clinical and radiographic parameters that distinguish between the best and worst outcomes of scoliosis surgery for adults. Eur Spine J. 2013;22:402–10.

66. Smith JS, Shaffrey CI, Lafage V, et al. Comparison of the best versus worst clinical outcomes for adult spinal deformity surgery: a retrospective review of a prospectively collected, multicenter database with 2-year follow-up. J Neurosurg Spine. 2015;23:349–59.

67. Smith JS, Singh M, Klineberg E, et al. Surgical treatment of pathological loss of lumbar lordosis (flatback) in the setting of normal sagittal vertical axis (SVA) achieves similar clinical improvement as surgical treatment of elevated SVA. J Neurosurg Spine. 2014;21:160–70.
68. Sethi R, Yanamadala V, Burton D, Bess RS. Using lean process improvement to enhance safety and value in orthopedic surgery: the case of spine surgery. J Am Acad Orthop Surg. 2017;25(11):E244–50.
69. Irwin Z, Hilibrand A, Gustavel M, et al. Variation in surgical decision making for degenerative spinal disorders. Part I: lumbar spine. Spine. 2005;30(19):2208–13.
70. Irwin Z, Hilibrand A, Gustavel M, et al. Variation in surgical decision making for degenerative spinal disorders. Part II: cervical spine. Spine. 2005;30(19):2214–9.
71. Madigosky W, van Schaik S. Context matters: groupthink and outcomes of health care teams. Med Educ. 2016;50:380–97.
72. Kana A, Wishart I, Fraser K, Coderre S, McLaughlin K. Are we at risk of groupthink in our approach to teamwork interventions in health care? Med Educ. 2016;50:400–8.
73. Mannion R, Thompson C. Systematic biases in group decision-making: implications for patient safety. Int J Qual Health Care. 2014;26(6):606–12.
74. Wolf M, Krause J, Carney P, Bogart A, Kurvers R. Collective intelligence meets medical decision-making: the collective outperforms the best radiologist. PLoS One. 2015;10(8):e0134269.
75. Kurvers RHJM, Herzog SM, Hertwig R, et al. Boosting medical diagnostics by pooling independent judgments. Proc Natl Acad Sci U S A. 2016;113(31):8777–82.
76. Weinstein JN. The missing piece: embracing shared decision making to reform health care. Spine (Phila Pa 1976). 2000;25(1):1–4.
77. Bonabeau E, Dorigo M, Theraulaz G. Swarm intelligence: from natural to artificial systems. Oxford: Oxford University Press; 1999.
78. Surowiecki J. The wisdom of crowds. New York: Anchor; 2005.
79. Couzin ID. Collective cognition in animal groups. Trends Cogn Sci. 2009;13:36–43.
80. Krause J, Ruxton GD, Krause S. Swarm intelligence in animals and humans. Trends Ecol Evol. 2010;25:28–34.
81. Mailoo V. Common sense or cognitive bias and groupthink: does it belong in our clinical reasoning? Br J Gen Pract. 2015;65(630):27.

The Seattle Spine Team Approach

Jean-Christophe A. Leveque

Deployment of system-wide continuous improvement strategies based on the fundamental principles of Lean methodology have been shown to result in fewer reoperations and a significant decrease in common perioperative adverse events [1]. While the theoretical framework behind Lean management was originally developed to eliminate deficiency and waste in the manufacturing industry; during the past decade or more, several healthcare institutions have implemented Lean and Six Sigma tools in their clinical practice [2–10]. An excellent example of Lean-based process improvement in healthcare was recently provided by Valentine and Falk who identified Toyota Production Systems' seven areas of waste (Fig. 6.1) in an anaesthesiology setting (Table 6.1) [7]. In the case of spine surgery, successful adaptation of Lean methodology by the Seattle Spine Team was recently described in detail by Sethi and colleagues [1, 9]. The Seattle Spine Team Model was designed as a three-pronged collaborative approach to the treatment of complex spinal deformity patients, utilizing a preoperative multidisciplinary

J.-C. A. Leveque (✉)
Neuroscience Institute, Virginia Mason Medical Center, Seattle, WA, USA

Department of Neurosurgery, Virginia Mason Medical Center, Seattle, WA, USA
e-mail: Jean-Christophe.Leveque@virginiamason.org

© Springer Nature Switzerland AG 2020
R. K. Sethi et al. (eds.), *Value-Based Approaches to Spine Care*,
https://doi.org/10.1007/978-3-030-31946-5_6

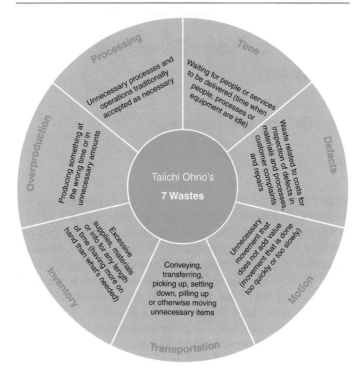

Fig. 6.1 Toyota Production System Seven Wastes. (©Virginia Mason Medical Center)

decision-making conference, a standardized intraoperative protocol for managing coagulopathy administered by a dedicated anesthesia team, and the mandated use of two attending surgeons [1, 11]. This combination led to a reduction in 30-day postoperative complications, although there was no observed difference in long-term outcomes between the pre- and post-protocol study groups. This chapter was designed to discuss the development of this type of protocol rather than merely rehash the specifics present within the initial publication. Our expectation is that this summary would provide the reader with

Table 6.1 Examples of types of waste identified in lean methodology

Type of waste	Description	Examples in anesthesia and spine surgery
Defect	Waste related to costs for inspection of defects in materials and processes, not meeting specifications	Medication errors
		Unplanned readmissions due to complications
Overproduction	Producing something at the wrong time or in unnecessary amounts	Unused blood products
		Unused sterile equipment
Waiting/time	Waiting for people or services to be delivered (people, processes or equipment are idle)	Waiting on laboratory results
		Waiting for operating room turnover
		Waiting for an available bed in PACU
Transportation	Conveying, transferring, picking up, setting down, piling up, or otherwise moving unnecessary items	Poor layout in patient flow leading to multiple patient transfers
Inventory	Supplies, material, or information exceeding what is required/needed	Unused sterile equipment
		Excessive stock in storerooms
Motion	Unnecessary movement performed too quickly or slowly, which does not add value to a process	Less than optimal operating room design resulting in unnecessary movement
		Unknown location of a needed item
Extra processing	Unnecessary processes and operations	Repeated collection of data, including laboratory testing, resulting in duplicate entries

Adapted from Valentine and Falk [7]; with permission

the understanding and tools necessary to design, develop, and implement such a protocol within any hospital system, as well as the justification for the involvement of relevant nonsurgical providers who may currently be involved in the care of these patients in a non-standardized manner.

Preoperative

The Seattle Spine Team protocol is initiated once the patient with a diagnosis of Adult Spinal Deformity (ASD) is scheduled for a consultation at our tertiary referral surgical spine clinic. The first step in the treatment pathway entails gathering a standard set of full-length scoliosis films needed to evaluate the extent of spino-pelvic malalignment as measured by sagittal and coronal balance, pelvic parameters, and Cobb angles of major and minor curves [12]. If symptoms of radiculopathy or neurogenic claudication are present on examination, Magnetic Resonance Imaging (MRI) of the lumbar spine is added to rule out disc herniation or spinal stenosis. Dual-energy x-ray absorptiometry (DEXA) measurements from the femoral neck are also collected in advance of a multidisciplinary case review to aid in the discussion of patient's risk for developing a non-union or Proximal Junction Kyphosis (PJK) following multilevel fusion for the correction of ASD [13–15]. Cohort studies have suggested that the risk of non-union and graft subsidence increases with a decreasing T-score [16], with similar findings reported by investigators analyzing the relationship between preoperative Vitamin D levels and postoperative outcomes following spine surgery [13–15]. Thus, we currently include femoral neck T-score measurements when assessing surgical appropriateness during patient's preoperative evaluation and counseling.

In addition to the radiographic data, we collect a comprehensive medical history and conduct a thorough physical examination for all patients with significant medical comorbidities and those who are expected to undergo a procedure involving six or more levels of fusion or six or more hours of case duration. A comprehensive report summarizing the patient and including preoperative Body Mass Index (BMI), age, Hemoglobin A1c [17–19], tobacco use, mental health [20–29], opioid utilization, pulmonary [30] and cardiac function [31], and radiographic data is prepared for presentation to a live multidisciplinary team consisting of neurosurgeons, dedicated complex spine anesthesiologists, orthopedic surgeons, internists, physiatrists, mental health professionals, and nurses as part of a comprehensive strategy aimed at preoperative risk mitigation.

Treatment recommendation provided by this core team of specialists is case-specific and evidence-based when possible. We understand that not all medical decisions can be supported by clear scientific evidence, and therefore we will attempt to reach a consensus opinion that balances our understanding of the relevant literature with the expertise and experience of the members of the conference. We attempt to allow for an equal "vote" by all team members independent of specialty and, in cases of significant dispute, we will attempt to identify particular areas of contention that could be addressed with further evaluation, a second opinion visit with a surgical or non-surgical provider, or further discussion with the patient. Documented recommendations are communicated to the patient at a follow-up visit and may involve additional testing or lifestyle modifications. Recognizing functional limitations, patients with BMI exceeding 40 kg/m^2 are counseled on potential lifestyle interventions and medical alternatives targeting weight loss, while patients with history of tobacco use and positive cotinine studies are offered various smoking cessation strategies well in advance of their scheduled surgery. The benefit of preoperative smoking cessation in patients undergoing surgery has been shown to correlate with the timing of the intervention, with greatest reduction in the rate of intra- and postoperative complications reported for patients whose smoking interventions were initiated at least 3 weeks before surgery [32, 33]. In our practice, two negative cotinine studies are required in patients with history of tobacco use with the second test scheduled at least 1 week prior to the schedule surgery. In the event of a positive test and after discussion with the patient, the surgical date will be rescheduled to allow for complete smoking cessation.

Results of non-surgical interventions and further diagnostic testing are re-presented on case-by-case basis at the monthly multidisciplinary conference. Upon consensus regarding surgical appropriateness, a tailored treatment plan is designed to provide optimal surgical correction while anticipating unavoidable patient-specific medical issues. For example, acute pain management of patients on active opioid replacement or agonist therapy prior to surgery due to history of addiction is provided by the dedicated Complex Spine Anesthesia Pain Service (APS). Faced with a complicated task of providing adequate pain relief in a patient population at a high risk of relapse [34], the APS team is essential to optimizing postoperative outcomes with a safe pain medication regimen.

Once cleared for surgery, a monthly educational class taught by a clinical nurse specialist offers another opportunity for patients and their caregivers to review surgical risks and procedure-related information. Administration of a health literacy questionnaire in the beginning of the class ensures that all learning styles and barriers to understanding are adequately addressed during both the class and following surgery. Previous studies have shown that patients who have limited comprehension of surgical risks are more like to be dissatisfied and file legal claims after surgery, while those who receive additional preoperative education report increased patient and family member satisfaction, fewer pain medication requests, and reduced length of hospital stay [35–38]. Since the clinical nurse specialist teaching the course is involved throughout the continuum of spine care, including in the preoperative multidisciplinary conference and postoperative outpatient care in the spine clinic, their experience facilitates ongoing communication with patients that can help clarify any points of misunderstanding or concern.

The final preoperative step is a preoperative clinic assessment by an anesthesiologist. This assessment is part of the standard work processes for any patient undergoing surgery at our institution, not only the complex spine patients, and the findings from this system review are used in standard OR work on the day of surgery.

Intraoperative

The intraoperative surgical plan will have been discussed and reviewed as part of the preoperative conference. During these discussions, the surgeons will review the rationale for the magnitude of the surgical procedure including the extent of fusion, the use of interbodies, the desired surgical goals, and the potential role for staging within the surgical procedure. The field of spine surgery is an ever-changing one, and we attempt to utilize current best practices in deciding upon the answers to the above questions. As discussed within the preoperative subsection, all patients will have a set of full-length standing scoliosis films and during the conference the type of deformity will be clearly identified. Our population is primarily an adult one, with a smaller subset of pediatric patients or adult patients with untreated adolescent curves, and so we will ensure that the surgical plan attempts to address issues of coronal and sagittal balance in addition to the more standard issues of central or foraminal stenosis that plague adult patients. Over the past decade, we have moved towards a greater use of lateral interbodies in the mid-lumbar levels or anterior interbodies at the lower lumbar levels to aid in lordosis restoration and eventual fusion. The decision for particular interbodies often guides the decision for staging of the surgical procedure. Our general algorithm is that any two surgical approaches can be performed within a single day, but if three distinct approaches are going to be utilized, then the operation will typically be staged over two separate days. In the earlier implementation of this protocol, the stages would be separated by 2–3 days to allow for some delayed resuscitation, but with greater experience of both the surgical and anesthesia teams, the two stages will typically be performed on sequential days. The anesthesia team typically will place a central line prior to any complex spine procedure with an expected blood loss approaching 1 L, which includes the majority of the scoliosis deformity procedures. In the event of a staged procedure we will aim to stack the interbody procedures on the first day to provide a large amount of the curve correction and indirect decompression. As these procedures are often performed through minimally invasive means or through smaller incisions that do not require extensive dissection, the central line is not placed on this first operative day but is instead placed after induction on the second day of surgery, thereby reducing the number of days that patients have an indwelling line. We understand that the data regarding surgical staging is conflicting [39–42], with some reports suggesting an increase in infection rates or total blood loss while other reports do not demonstrate such effects. In our experience, the potential advantage of completing an operative procedure involving three approaches within one operative setting are outweighed by the length of the surgical day, the fatigue of the operative team, the potential requirement upon substitute operating room personnel in the late afternoon or early evening hours, and the development of an intraoperative coagulopathy that appears to be time-related. This late coagulopathy can drive up the blood loos in later portions of the surgical procedure and further slow the operating team as they struggle to complete the procedure in an operative field that is partially obscured by ongoing bleeding. This staging decision is one that will have to be made by each individual surgical/anesthesia team, and we agree that others may place a lesser or greater reliance on the use of alternate approaches for the placement of interbodies that may lead to different decisions regarding the role for operative staging. We would hasten to add, however, that it has also been our experience that including the option for staging and not requiring it due to an easier-than-expected procedure is often far better received than the opposite, and therefore especially in the younger surgeon's or newer teams' career, such an option should be srongly considered.

The Seattle Spine Team Approach mandates the use of two surgeons for complex spine procedures. The logic behind this portion of the protocol arose from the airline industry's use of pilot-copilot roles for all larger carrier airplanes. The medical community has recognized that there may be benefit to utilizng the learnings of other industries that have instruments of high complexity and which involve the direct care of human life [43]. Operator error is a potentially controllable source of poor outcome, and the presence of a surgical colleague may be able to reduce this risk. This colleague can aid not only the physical component of the surgical work, but can aid in decision-making during the procedure. In the case of a straightforward uncomplicated case, the mental load of surgery may be relatively minimal, but the field of complex spine surgery is often filled with less than ideal situations, including abnormal anatomy, unclear boundaries, or previous scar and the loss of standard landmarks. These difficult scenarios may be surmounted more easily with two proficient surgeons than one. The effect of the two-surgeon model has been studied in both adult and pediatric spine surgery [44–46], with most studies demonstrating an improvement in both operative time and total estimated blood loss and some describing a reduction in surgical complications. While the question may arise as to the need for two attending surgeons versus merely one attending and an experienced fellow, one study that broke down the surgical procedure into six individual steps noted a significant improvement in operative time in four of these steps when two attendings were used rather than an attending and fellow [46]. Our initial protocol called specifically for two attending surgeons, however with the greater experience of the surgical team and in the presence of a fellow with appropriate surgical skills, we allow for completion of a surgical case by an attending and fellow after discussion with the anesthesia team and other attending surgeons. More difficult procedures such as pedicle subtraction osteotomies, severe revision cases or more pronounced deformities are still performed by two attending surgeons, however. This requirement does have financial and scheduling ramifications, and it appears that the difficulty in implementing this portion of the protocol in other institutions is primarily related to these two factors, even as many surgeons agree with its benefits [47].

The operating room environment has also been standardized to improve efficiency in room setup time, movement throughout the room during the case, and easier identification of any missing or misplaced operating room equipment. The complex spine cases take place within a specified operating room and on dedicated operative days rather than added on to the operating room schedule in any available room, also minimizing the chaos that might otherwise go along with re-creating this setup in different rooms on different days. Over time, this room setup was codified into a "room map" that functions as a checklist at the start of the operative day to ensure that all elements are present (Fig. 6.2). This room map will necessarily change over time as operating rooms are updated or newer equipment is purchased, but even the presence of such a map can aid in determining what is feasible when making these purchasing, moving, or renovating decisions.

The anesthesia team maintains a standardized intraoperative protocol that addresses all aspects of anesthesia care during the surgical procedure. The protocol goes through the surgical

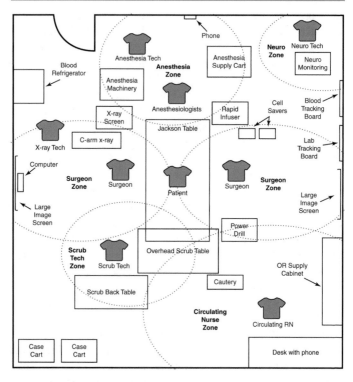

Fig. 6.2 Standard operating room layout for a complex spine procedure. The layout is designed to have dedicated zones of operation for the surgeons and scrub technicians, circulating nurse, anesthesia team, and neuromonitoring team. Radiologic studies can be seen on two large-image screens placed on opposite walls. Neuro Tech indicates neurological technician, Neuro monitoring neurological monitoring, Scrub Tech scrub technician, OR operating room, RN registered nurse. (Adapted from Sethi et al. [1]; with permission)

procedure in a stepwise fashion, noting medications to be used for induction, maintenaince, and awakening that are specifically chosen to allow for appropriate neuromonitoring during spinal surgery. The protocol describes standard timepoints for lab checks and the normal lab values as well as specific changes that might require intervention. This written protocol is kept online and updated quarterly. Any new team member or resident rotating onto the service is provided access to this online version and is expected to have read it prior to the procedure. This easily accessible online document helps ensure that all members are following best practices and minimizes the Given the potential for high blood loss during these cases, blood products are ordered preoperatively and delivered to the room at the start of the case. These products are kept within a blood refrigerator in the room, and as products are administrated their use is tracked visually on a dry-erase board mounted on the wall so that the entire surgical team can at any moment have an immediate assessment of the blood loss and the resuscitative efforts.

The advantages of a team-based coordinated approach can be seen in the ease of implementing marginal change over time. At the start of our Seattle Spine Team Approach in 2010, the typical blood products ordered for a complex spine case included 6 units of packed red blood cells and 4 units of fresh frozen plasma (FFP). With the growing evidence for the use of tranexamic acid (TXA) in complex spine surgery, we have included an assessment of a patient's appropriateness for this medication as a part of our preoperative conference since mid-2015. The combination of TXA and an increased reliance on lateral or anterior approaches for interbody placement has led to an overall decrease in the total EBL for these procedures, which now typically are performed with less than 1000cc rather than the 1500–2500cc blood loss that was more common in the 2010–2014 era. Noting this decreased EBL over time, the anesthesia team was able to quickly implement a reduction in the pre-ordered blood products for each case thereby decreasing the waste of unused blood and FFP. This implementation was facilitated by the pre-existing loci for communication, including the monthly complex spine conference and the quarterly anesthesia complex spine team meeting. An update to the online document after discussion with team members meant that the change could be easily dispersed to all necessary parties and enacted rapidly.

Conclusion

The success of any operative procedure is often felt to rely upon the skill and expertise of the primary surgeon. Patients typically seek out specific individuals for their surgical care, whereas the same often does not hold true for specialized medical care. When faced with a complex medical problem or cancer care, patients often will choose a medical *system* for their treatment, understanding that the coordination of multiple specialties may be required to obtain optimal outcomes. Historically the allure of the "top surgeon", however, has held sway and is even promoted in popular television and media portrayals. This concept nowadays may be an illusion, however, as clearly an individual surgeon is no more able to carry an operation through to its successful result without any assistance than an airline pilot would be able to fly an airliner without a ground crew, support staff, and traffic control personnel. Indeed, as we within surgical fields have recently looked to the airline industry for guidance in the development of medical checklists and standardization, the analogy sustains.

When faced with the treatment of complex conditions such as adolescent and adult degenerative scoliosis, therefore, it may be foolhardy to believe that the individual surgeon can serve as the dictator and final arbiter for all of the events that surround a potential operative candidate's care. When we consider the breadth of advances in the treatment of scoliosis over the last decade and the difficulty even we as surgeons have in keeping abreast of these advances, it is unreasonable to assume that any one individual can maintain updated proficiency in anesthetic medications, hypertensive treatments, cardiac pre-clearance, and the myriad issues that may go into the pre-, intra- and post-operative treatment of a surgical patient. By necessity, we delegate authority to our colleagues in associated specialties and rely on their knowledge of the most up-to-date interventions that might provide best outcomes, and we generally question their judgement only when their proposals contradict our understanding of the current medical situation or some of our long-held but sometimes outdated historical body of medical knowledge. Yet it is in this delegation of responsibility that the potential for error or misunderstanding may arise. When asked, many patients seem to believe that we within the medical system have a universal medical record that all providers can access, so that we are each able to fully understand the full depth and breadth of a patient's preoperative history and the results of individual tests and interventions. Within the United States, however, such as a system is essentially a myth, and we therefore rely on incomplete records cobbled together from disparate providers, sometimes over great spans of time and distance. When the operative date arises, therefore, while a patient and their family may believe that the primary care doctor who provided preoperative clearance has an intimate knowledge of the proposed surgical procedure, and that the surgical anesthesiologist for the day has spoken directly to both the primary care doctor and the surgeon about the plan of care for the operation and the days beyond, and that the surgeon and her team will transition the patient's care from the hospital setting back to their home community with grace, the truth typically lies far from this utopian ideal.

The purpose of the above paragraphs is not to malign the current medical system, but rather to attempt to provide an honest assessment of the difficulties that we face when treating complex surgical conditions and therefore lay out the argument for a standardized and coordinated team to address potential issues throughout all phases of surgical care. At its essence, the purpose of the Seattle Spine Team Approach and other such protocols is to provide a framework for all providers that care for these patients which can identify areas of concern that might, if left untreated or unassessed, lead to complications or unintended outcomes that reduce the efficacy and safety of our interventions. It is clear that many surgeons have been able to create individualized systems that maintain a high degree of success with very low complication rates without the support of a large standardized team approach. Rather than rely on the ability of a particular surgeons to create such a system de novo in each specific hospital system, however, it may be more prudent to develop specific team-based pathways for surgical success that can be translated from institution to institution. If the positive effects of these team-based approaches can be demonstrated scientifically, then these results may serve as an impetus for a hospital or medical system to support the creation and maintenance of team pathways. Such external support is often required when one considers the time and effort required from individual providers from disparate specialties, and especially when one assesses the specific details such as a meeting space and time, administrative and/or technical support, and the ability to record and study the results of these interventions within the medical record.

When assessing any particular protocol, the question of its origin is often helpful to understand the defects that the pathway aims to address. In our case of the Seattle Spine Team Approach, our "stop-the-line" moment came after a patient death during a pedicle subtraction osteotomy. Virginia Mason Hospital utilized a Toyota model of LEAN approaches to the administration of health care throughout the hospital, but such a process is not critical to the development of a standardized approach to care. Rather, the presence of such a process aids in communicating the urgency to all involved parties and helps in assembling a team to address defects without a punitive focus. In our circumstance, when we assessed the pre- and intra-operative circumstances that surrounded this patient's death, a few obvious issues came to light. We also considered the complication of a postoperative hemorrhagic cerebellar stroke after scoliosis surgery in a patient 6 months earlier in our analysis, as it became clear that what at the time had seemed like an unexplained issue of coagulopathy might not actually have been a random event that was unlikely to be repeated.

The intraoperative events were the easiest to approach and understand for the surgical team: the operative start time, the surgeon team involved in the case, the experience of the anesthesia team with cases of this magnitude, the anesthetic medication choices, the effect of neuromonitoring on both the surgeons and the anesthesiologists, the use of intraoperative blood transfusion and the means of getting blood to the OR, and the possibility of any medication error during the more chaotic situation of an operating room rather than on a patient ward. It would have been simple, and even expected, for a review to focus on these entities and identify points of fault and then pass blame, prohibit such procedures in the future or put half-measures into place. Rather than pursue such a route, however, the reviewing team chose to spend time developing an operative protocol that would address each of these issues in a standardized manner. The anesthesiologists decided that cases of this magnitude should be approached in a manner similar to cardiac surgery, with a dedicated team that understood the interplay of anesthesia, neuromonitoring, and potential for high blood loss and could continue to work together over time to refine specific protocol interventions. Although it was relatively common practice to have two surgeons performing these more complex cases, the protocol made such practice required, which served not only to allow for appropriate scheduling but also was an indicator to the hospital system that the presence of two surgeons was a safety measure, not merely one of surgeon desire or preference. Numerous other small interventions were included to address other potential intraoperative sources of error or misjudgment.

Interestingly, the reviewing team in this case also sought to understand the route that these patients took in their clinical path to the operating room. Questions were asked about this patient and future patients' suitability for surgery of this magnitude, and since in this cases care was coordinated between an independent medical system and the hospital itself, how could one ensure that all of the required information had been passed to all relevant parties? The initial proposal for a preoperative multidisciplinary conference was largely aimed at assessing relevant areas of concern prior to surgery, predominantly within the cardiac and pulmonary realms. Over time, however, it has become clear that the presence of multiple experts in a room may allow for expansion beyond the simple question of preoperative readiness, and can instead allow for exploration of alternate treatments or lesser invasive surgical options, especially when adjunct fields to spine treatment such as anesthesia pain and physiatry are included.

This concept of a multidisciplinary team is not novel, at least within the field of medicine. Most hospitals have weekly or monthly tumor boards that span across surgical and medical disciplines and are designed to address the ideal personalized treatment for patients depending on an analysis of history, radiographic findings, pathology specimens, and expectations of outcome [48]. Many such meetings have set protocols to ensure that newer treatments or studies are considered, and most suggest that an ideal makeup of participants requires members from all relevant fields for the particular disease under consideration. When one considers the Seattle Spine Team preoperative conference in such a light, its existence is perhaps a little less novel, although perhaps its use as a preoperative decision-making conference in a historically independent field such as spine surgery makes it so. Some surgeons have raised concerns that this type of conference impedes on a surgeon's independence or supposes that surgeons are incapable of identifying appropriate patients for surgery or of recognizing preoperative factors that might predispose to poorer outcomes. To these objections, we would counter that we hope to achieve the same goals that are sought by a tumor board: the best individualized treatment for each patient taking into account the full range of their medical history combined with the potential surgical and nonsurgical skills of the treating team.

References

1. Sethi RK, Pong RP, Leveque J-C, Dean TC, Olivar SJ, Rupp SM. The Seattle Spine Team approach to adult deformity surgery: a systems-based approach to perioperative care and subsequent reduction in perioperative complication rates. Spine Deform. 2014;2(2):95–103.
2. Womack JP, Womack JP, Jones DT, Roos D. Machine that changed the world. New York, New York: Simon and Schuster; 1990.
3. Idemoto L, Williams B, Blackmore C. Using lean methodology to improve efficiency of electronic order set maintenance in the hospital. BMJ Open Qual. 2016;5(1):u211725. w4724.
4. Cima RR, Brown MJ, Hebl JR, Moore R, Rogers JC, Kollengode A, et al. Use of lean and six sigma methodology to improve operating room efficiency in a high-volume tertiary-care academic medical center. J Am Coll Surg. 2011;213(1):83–92.
5. Blackmore CG, Kaplan GS. Lean and the perfect patient experience. BJM Quality and Safety. 2017;26:85–86.
6. Ferguson A, Uldall K, Dunn J, Blackmore CC, Williams B. Effectiveness of a multifaceted delirium screening, prevention, and treatment initiative on the rate of delirium falls in the acute care setting. J Nurs Care Qual. 2018;33(3):213–20.

7. Valentine EA, Falk SA. Quality improvement in anesthesiology—leveraging data and analytics to optimize outcomes. Anesthesiol Clin. 2018;36(1):31–44.

8. Kim CS, Spahlinger DA, Kin JM, Billi JE. Lean health care: what can hospitals learn from a world-class automaker? J Hosp Med. 2006;1(3):191–9.

9. Sethi R, Yanamadala V, Burton DC, Bess RS. Using lean process improvement to enhance safety and value in orthopaedic surgery: the case of spine surgery. J Am Acad Orthop Surg (JAAOS). 2017;25(11):e244–e50.

10. Wellman J, Jeffries H, Hagan P. Leading the lean healthcare journey: driving culture change to increase value. Portland: CRC Press; 2016.

11. Buchlak QD, Yanamadala V, Leveque J-C, Sethi R. Complication avoidance with pre-operative screening: insights from the Seattle spine team. Curr Rev Musculoskelet Med. 2016;9(3):316–26.

12. Schwab F, Ungar B, Blondel B, Buchowski J, Coe J, Deinlein D, et al. Scoliosis Research Society—Schwab adult spinal deformity classification: a validation study. Spine. 2012;37(12):1077–82.

13. Schofferman J, Schofferman L, Zucherman J, Hsu K, White A. Metabolic bone disease in lumbar pseudarthrosis. Spine. 1990;15(7):687–9.

14. Ravindra VM, Godzik J, Dailey AT, Schmidt MH, Bisson EF, Hood RS, et al. Vitamin D levels and 1-year fusion outcomes in elective spine surgery. Spine. 2015;40(19):1536–41.

15. Kerezoudis P, Rinaldo L, Drazin D, Kallmes D, Krauss W, Hassoon A, et al. Association between vitamin D deficiency and outcomes following spinal fusion surgery: a systematic review. World Neurosurg. 2016;95:71–6.

16. Tempel ZJ, Gandhoke GS, Okonkwo DO, Kanter AS. Impaired bone mineral density as a predictor of graft subsidence following minimally invasive transpsoas lateral lumbar interbody fusion. Eur Spine J. 2015;24(3):414–9.

17. Walid MS, Newman BF, Yelverton JC, Nutter JP, Ajjan M, Robinson JS Jr. Prevalence of previously unknown elevation of glycosylated hemoglobin in spine surgery patients and impact on length of stay and total cost. J Hosp Med. 2010;5(1):E10–E4.

18. Takahashi S, Suzuki A, Toyoda H, Terai H, Dohzono S, Yamada K, et al. Characteristics of diabetes associated with poor improvements in clinical outcomes after lumbar spine surgery. Spine. 2013;38(6):516–22.

19. Hikata T, Iwanami A, Hosogane N, Watanabe K, Ishii K, Nakamura M, et al. High preoperative hemoglobin A1c is a risk factor for surgical site infection after posterior thoracic and lumbar spinal instrumentation surgery. J Orthop Sci. 2014;19(2):223–8.

20. Hägg O, Fritzell P, Ekselius L, Nordwall A. Predictors of outcome in fusion surgery for chronic low back pain. A report from the Swedish Lumbar Spine Study. Eur Spine J. 2003;12(1):22–33.

21. Parker SL, Chaichana KL, Mukherjee D, Adogwa O, Cheng J, McGirt M. Correlation of preoperative depression and somatic perception scales with postoperative disability and quality of life after lumbar discectomy. Spine J. 2010;10(9):S16–S7.

22. Adogwa O, Parker SL, Shau DN, Mendenhall SK, Aaronson OS, Cheng JS, et al. Preoperative Zung Depression Scale predicts outcome after revision lumbar surgery for adjacent segment disease, recurrent stenosis, and pseudarthrosis. Spine J. 2012;12(3):179–85.

23. Carr FA, Healy KM, Villavicencio AT, Nelson EL, Mason A, Burneikiene S, et al. Effect on clinical outcomes of patient pain expectancies and preoperative mental component summary scores from the 36-item short form health survey following anterior cervical discectomy and fusion. J Neurosurg Spine. 2011;15(5):486–90.

24. Bakhsheshian J, Scheer JK, Gum JL, Hostin R, Lafage V, Bess S, et al. Impact of poor mental health in adult spinal deformity patients with poor physical function: a retrospective analysis with a 2-year follow-up. J Neurosurg Spine. 2017;26(1):116–24.

25. Diebo BG, Lavian JD, Murray DP, Liu S, Shah NV, Beyer GA, et al. The impact of comorbid mental health disorders on complications following adult spinal deformity surgery with minimum 2-year surveillance. Spine. 2018;43(17):1176–83.

26. Shah I, Wang C, Jain N, Formanek B, Buser Z, Wang JC. Postoperative complications in adult spinal deformity patients with a mental illness undergoing reconstructive thoracic or thoracolumbar spine surgery. Spine J. 2019;19:662–9.

27. Adogwa O, Verla T, Thompson P, Penumaka A, Kudyba K, Johnson K, et al. Affective disorders influence clinical outcomes after revision lumbar surgery in elderly patients with symptomatic adjacent-segment disease, recurrent stenosis, or pseudarthrosis. J Neurosurg Spine. 2014;21(2):153–9.

28. Trief PM, Ploutz-Snyder R, Fredrickson BE. Emotional health predicts pain and function after fusion: a prospective multicenter study. Spine. 2006;31(7):823–30.

29. Menendez ME, Neuhaus V, Bot AG, Ring D, Cha TD. Psychiatric disorders and major spine surgery: epidemiology and perioperative outcomes. Spine. 2014;39(2):E111–E22.

30. Jackson RP, Simmons E, Stripinis D. Coronal and sagittal plane spinal deformities correlating with back pain and pulmonary function in adult idiopathic scoliosis. Spine. 1989;14(12):1391–7.

31. Eagle KA, Berger PB, Calkins H, Chaitman BR, Ewy GA, Fleischmann KE, et al. ACC/AHA guideline update for perioperative cardiovascular evaluation for noncardiac surgery—executive summary: a report of the American College of Cardiology/American Heart Association task force on practice guidelines (committee to update the 1996 guidelines on perioperative cardiovascular evaluation for noncardiac surgery). J Am Coll Cardiol. 2002;39(3):542–53.

32. Møller AM, Villebro N, Pedersen T, Tønnesen H. Effect of preoperative smoking intervention on postoperative complications: a randomised clinical trial. Lancet. 2002;359(9301):114–7.

33. Nakagawa M, Tanaka H, Tsukuma H, Kishi Y. Relationship between the duration of the preoperative smoke-free period and the incidence of post-

operative pulmonary complications after pulmonary surgery. Chest. 2001;120(3):705–10.

34. Bryson EO. The perioperative management of patients maintained on medications used to manage opioid addiction. Curr Opin Anaesthesiol. 2014;27(3):359–64.

35. Vincent C, Phillips A, Young M. Why do people sue doctors? A study of patients and relatives taking legal action. Lancet. 1994;343(8913):1609–13.

36. Huntington B, Kuhn N, editors. Communication gaffes: a root cause of malpractice claims. Baylor University Medical Center Proceedings. Taylor & Francis; 2003.

37. Yoon RS, Nellans KW, Geller JA, Kim AD, Jacobs MR, Macaulay W. Patient education before hip or knee arthroplasty lowers length of stay. J Arthroplast. 2010;25(4):547–51.

38. Kruzik N. Benefits of preoperative education for adult elective surgery patients. AORN J. 2009;90(3):381–7.

39. Passias PG, Poorman GW, Jalai CM, Line B, Diebo B, Park P, et al. Outcomes of open staged corrective surgery in the setting of adult spinal deformity. Spine J. 2017;17(8):1091–9.

40. Rhee JM, Bridwell KH, Lenke LG, Baldus C, Blanke K, Edwards C, et al. Staged posterior surgery for severe adult spinal deformity. Spine. 2003;28(18):2116–21.

41. Maddox JJ, Pruitt DR, Agel J, Bransford RJ. Unstaged versus staged posterior-only thoracolumbar fusions in deformity: a retrospective comparison of perioperative complications. Spine J. 2014;14(7):1159–65.

42. Gum JL, Lenke LG, Bumpass D, Zhao J, Sugrue P, Karikari I, et al. Does planned staging for posterior-only vertebral column resections in spinal deformity surgery increase perioperative complications? Spine Deform. 2016;4(2):131–7.

43. Helmreich RL. On error management: lessons from aviation. BMJ. 2000;320(7237):781–5.

44. Gomez J, Lafage V, Sciubba DM, Bess S, Mundis GM, Liabaud B, et al. Adult scoliosis deformity (ASD) surgery: comparison of one versus two attending surgeons' clinical outcomes. Spine J. 2015;15(10):S156.

45. Halanski MA, Elfman CM, Cassidy JA, Hassan NE, Sund SA, Noonan KJ. Comparing results of posterior spine fusion in patients with AIS: are two surgeons better than one? J Orthop. 2013;10(2):54–8.

46. Chan CYW, Kwan MK. Perioperative outcome in posterior spinal fusion for adolescent idiopathic scoliosis: a prospective study comparing single versus two attending surgeons strategy. Spine. 2016;41(11):E694–E9.

47. Scheer JK, Hey L, Lagrone M, Daubs M, Ames CP. 343 results of the 2015 SRS survey on single versus two attending surgeon approach for adult spinal deformity surgery. Neurosurgery. 2016;63:201.

48. Newman EA, Guest AB, Helvie MA, Roubidoux MA, Chang AE, Kleer CG, et al. Changes in surgical management resulting from case review at a breast cancer multidisciplinary tumor board. Cancer. 2006;107(10):2346–51.

Modifiable Factors in a Standard Work Protocol for Adult Deformity Surgery

7

Douglas C. Burton

The incidence of adult spinal deformity (ASD) continues to increase with our aging population [1]. As baby boomers age, their expectations and desire for medical interventions to improve and lengthen their quality of life have put unprecedented pressure on spine care professionals. At the same time, surgeries not considered possible or reasonable 20 years ago are now being performed on a regular basis [2]. Improvement in the quality of life in this patient population can be exceedingly high; a large percentage of the patients report satisfaction with their surgery and its outcome [3]. Unfortunately, the complication rate of ASD surgery also remains incredibly high, with up to 70% of the patients experiencing some type of a complication, as described in the largest published series in the literature [4].

The confluence of an aging population with unprecedented health expectations and improved technology to deliver increasing complex care to older individuals, coupled with a high complication rate, have created an economic crisis in this arena of medicine. The cost of delivering this care is not sustainable, particularly when the cost of complications is added to the equation. As health economics research has focused on this problem and

D. C. Burton (✉)
Department of Orthopaedic Surgery, Kansas City Medical Center, Kansas City, KS, USA
e-mail: dburton@kumc.edu

© Springer Nature Switzerland AG 2020
R. K. Sethi et al. (eds.), *Value-Based Approaches to Spine Care*,
https://doi.org/10.1007/978-3-030-31946-5_7

this patient population, several facts have emerged. The cost of implants and biologics make up a large percentage of the direct cost of care; however, it is the cost of complications, particularly those that drive reoperation and readmission, that tips the value equation against these operations for these patients [5].

Some surgeons, understanding this dilemma, have implemented risk stratification algorithms for the patients they consider for surgery [6, 7]. They have shown improvements in outcomes and decrease in complications following a multidisciplinary evaluation of patients considered for surgery; however, critics of this approach claim this denial of care. While it is true that some patients are just not candidates for surgery, it is our belief that many may not currently be a candidate but could become one through health optimization.

Over the course of this chapter, we will discuss a series of modifiable factors that have been shown in the literature to impact complications, readmissions, and reoperations. Knowing that a factor makes a difference is not enough, however. To actually affect change, these individual optimizations have to be applied to every patient, every time in a consistent manner. This is the charge of standard work – breaking down a process into discrete steps, and then performing them in a consistent manner regardless of the operator [8]. The first nine are patient-specific factors that can be modified: albumin, smoking, bone mineral density (BMD), hemoglobin, body mass index (BMI), frailty, hemoglobin A1c, mental health, and vitamin D. While the last two are intraoperative and include employing spine-specific fluid management algorithms, or administering tranexamic acid.

Preoperative Patient Factors

Albumin

Albumin and prealbumin are serum proteins that have been recognized as markers for increased risk of complications in patients undergoing surgery. While normative values vary among laboratories, a typical adult serum albumin range is 3.5–5.0 g/dL, and between 20 and 36 mg/dL for circulating levels of prealbumin. Schoenfeld et al. queried the National Quality Improvement Program (NSQIP) for patients undergoing spinal arthrodesis surgery and found that more than two thousand patients had their preoperative albumin level collected [9]. Their study showed that preoperative albumin levels of 3.5 g/dL or lower were associated with an increased 13.8 odds ratio (OR) for mortality, a 2.5 OR for wound infection, and a threefold increase in complications.

Adogwa published two separate studies analyzing the correlation between serum albumin levels and complications and readmissions [10, 11]. In 2014, they studied 136 patients undergoing spine surgery and found that a serum albumin level under 3.5 g/dl was associated with a threefold increase in complications. The adjusted analysis also showed that a serum albumin level of 3.5 g/dL or less was independently associated with complications. In another report, Adogwa et al. demonstrated that of 145 patients who had undergone elective spine surgery, those who had serum albumin levels of less than 3.5 g/dL were likely to be readmitted.

Tempel et al. [12] found that among 83 patients treated for a postoperative wound infection after spine surgery, 82 had prealbumin levels below 20 mg/dL. Bohl et al. [13] studied 4310 NSQIP patients and found serum albumin level less than 3.5 g/dL was an independent risk factor for infections and wound complications, as well as 30-day readmissions and extended hospital stays. Finally, Fu et al. [14] queried the NSQIP database and showed an association between hypoalbuminemia and increased complications and inpatient stays in patients undergoing anterior cervical discectomy and fusion.

We currently use albumin and prealbumin tests as screening tools in our clinic. Any patient being considered for surgery who has low levels of either may is referred to our nutritionist or to their internist to work up the cause of these low levels (Table 7.1).

Smoking

The use of nicotine, particularly smoking, is known to cause a wide range of health problems, including lung cancer [15] and

Table 7.1 Preoperative – albumin and prealbumin

Author(s)	Study design	Evidence level	N (total)	Mean age, years ± SD; years (range)	Variable evaluated: serum albumin (g/dL)/Pre-albumin (mg/dL) cut-off value	Conclusion
Schoenfeld et al. [9]	Retrospective	III	5887	55.9 ± 14.5	3.5	Serum albumin level <3.5 g/dL was associated with increased mortality, complications, wound infection and thromboembolic disease
Adogwa et al. [10]	Retrospective	III	145	56.46 ± 13.64 (>3.6 g/dL) 58.90 ± 18.01 (≤3.5 g/dL)	3.5	Preoperative serum albumin level <3.5 g/dL was an independent predictor of 30-day readmission following elective spine surgery
Adogwa et al. [11]	Retrospective	III	136	53.8 ± 17.0	3.5	Preoperative serum albumin level <3.5 g/dL was an independent predictor of postoperative complications following elective spine surgery

Tempel et al. [12]	Retrospective	IV	83	56 (19–85)[a]	20	Serum prealbumin level <20 mg/dL may be associated with postoperative wound infection
Bohl et al. [13]	Retrospective	III	4310	N/A	3.5	Preoperative serum albumin level <3.5 g/dL was associated with increased rates of wound dehiscence, UTI, SSI, longer LOS, and 30-day unplanned RA
Fu et al. [14]	Retrospective	III	3671	52.2 ± 11.3	3.5	Preoperative serum albumin level <3.5 g/dL was an independent predictor of major postoperative complications.

Our current practice: any patient being considered for surgery who has low levels of albumin or prealbumin is referred to our nutritionist or to their internist to work up the cause of these low levels

[a]Available for patients who developed an infection

other forms of cancer [16]. Its association with adverse outcomes in adult spinal surgery and spinal deformity surgery has been demonstrated by several studies [17–23].

Soroceanu et al. [18] showed that smoking was associated with increased risk of medical complications in 448 patients who had undergone ASD surgery. In a population-based study of 35,477 patients undergoing lumbar spine surgery Martin et al. [19] demonstrated an increase in wound complications and higher incidence of 30-day morbidity in patients with a history of smoking.

Conflicting results have been published on the risks between reoperation and smoking. Mok et al. [22] and Puvanesarajah et al. [23] both found an association with reoperation in patients undergoing lumbar spine surgery. Scheer et al., on the other hand, did not find an association when evaluating 352 patients undergoing adult spinal deformity surgery.

Our current practice is to include nicotine use evaluation as part of our general diagnostic workup. If patients use nicotine products, we do not schedule them for surgery until they have completed nicotine cessation and have cotinine levels of nonsmokers (Table 7.2). Many patients can accomplish this on their own but some may need medications and/or support group assistance to accomplish this. Carlson et al. [24] have shown that the one-year recidivism is 60% with this approach. This is the same success rate of nicotine cessation seen by patients seeking to quit smoking of their own volition [25].

Bone Mineral Density

Several studies have looked at BMD and its association with complications. Three studies identified and association between decreased BMD and screw loosening in adult spinal surgery [26–28]. Okuyama et al. [26] found that decreased bone density was associated with pseudoarthrosis. In a large study of over 2200 patients in the Pearl Diver database, Puvanesaraja et al. [23] showed that osteoporosis was a significant predictor for revision surgery with an odds ratio (OR) of 1.98 ($p < 0.0001$).

Table 7.2 Preoperative – smoking

Author(s)	Study design	Evidence level	N (total)	Mean age, years ± SD; year (range)	Variable evaluated: smoking	Conclusion
Tang et al. [17]	Retrospective	IV	236	61.7 (47–77)	History of smoking (within 1 year of surgery) obtained from medical record	Smoking was not associated with postoperative complications following degenerative lumbar scoliosis surgery
Soroceanu et al. [18]	Retrospective	IV	448	56.8 (15.45)	Smoking history obtained from a multi-institutional database	Smoking was independently associated with postoperative complications following ASD surgery
Martin et al. [19]	Retrospective	IV	35,477	51 ± 13 (current) 64 ± 13 (former) 60 ± 15 (never)	Smoking status obtained from a multi-institutional database and categorized as never (no use), prior (quit more than 12 months before surgery), and current (within 1 year of surgery) smoker	Smoking status was independently associated with SSI, and 30-day morbidity following lumbar spine surgery

(continued)

Table 7.2 (continued)

Author(s)	Study design	Evidence level	N (total)	Mean age, years ± SD; year (range)	Variable evaluated: smoking	Conclusion
McCunniff et al. [20]	Retrospective	III	559	55.1 ± 13.5 (smoker cohort) 53.2 ± 16.8 (nonsmoker cohort)	Patient-reported smoking history in packs per day was obtained from medical records. Patient who continued smoking up until the day of surgery was defined as a smoker.	Smoking was independently associated with increased EBL, perioperative transfusion rate in patients undergoing lumbar spine surgery
Inoue et al. [21]	Retrospective	IV	76	62.4 ± 10.8	History of smoking obtained from medical record	Smoking was independently associated with critical mechanical failure following ASD surgery
Mok et al. [22]	Retrospective	IV	89	48.5 ± 15.5	History of smoking obtained from medical record. Patients smoking until the day of surgery were categorized as smokers	In adjusted analysis, smoking status was associated with ROR following primary ASD surgery
Puvanesarajah et al. [23]	Retrospective	IV	2293	65–84	History of smoking obtained from PearlDiver database	In adjusted analysis, smoking was an independent predictor of ROR following posterolateral fusion of 8 or more levels (OR 1.37, 95% CI 1.10–1.70)

Our current practice: nicotine use is evaluate as part of general diagnostic workup. If patients use nicotine products, we do not schedule them for surgery until they have completed nicotine cessation and have cotinine levels of nonsmokers

Proximal junctional kyphosis (PJK) remains a common and vexing complication in ASD surgery. Three separate studies, including one meta-analysis [29] found an association between decreased BMD and PJK [29–31]. Liu et al. [29] identified three studies in the literature linking low BMD with an increased incidence of PJK. Yagi et al. [32] reported that female ASD patients treated with teriparatide immediately after surgery for ASD had improved volumetric bone density and less incidence of PJK (4.6% vs. 15.2%) when compared to controls.

Our current practice is to screen all preoperative patients with dual energy x-ray absorptiometry (DEXA). Any patient with a T score of less than −1.5 is started on teriparatide 20 micrograms subcutaneously daily for 3 months prior to surgery and then 3 months after surgery (Table 7.3). Our early results are promising. There is speculation that use of these medications may improve fusion rates, but this remains speculation and further study is needed to understand this potential benefit.

Preoperative Hemoglobin

There are a handful of studies that have shown an association between a low preoperative hemoglobin and complications and increased need for transfusion. Five studies [33–37] of over 26,000 total patients showed an association between low preoperative hemoglobin level and increased risk of major transfusion. Seican et al. [38] reviewed a large administrative database of 24,473 patients and found that patients with hematocrit graded as mild (30–37%) to severe (<26%) had increased major and minor complications, longer length of stay, and greater 30-day mortality compared to patients with no (>38%) anemia.

We currently refer all our patients with a hemoglobin of <12.0 g/dL (female) or <13.5 g/dL (males) to our blood management clinic. They perform a complete workup for causes of anemia and treat our patients as appropriate. We have made this a part of our standard work but have not been performing this long enough to evaluate our results (Table 7.4).

Table 7.3 Preoperative – bone mineral density (BMD)

Author(s)	Study design	Evidence level	N (total)	Mean age, years ± SD; year (range)	Variable evaluated: bone mineral density	Conclusion
Okuyama et al. [26]	Retrospective	III	52	63 (45–76)	Continuous BMD (g/cm²)	Decrease in BMD was associated with screw loosening and nonunion following pedicle screw fixation in conjunction with PLIF. Bone density of 0.674 ± 0.104 g/cm² was proposed as a threshold value
Puvanesarajah et al. [23]	Retrospective	III	2293	65–84	History of osteoporosis obtained from PearlDiver database	In adjusted analysis, osteoporosis was an independent predictor of ROR following posterolateral fusion of 8 or more levels (OR 1.98, 95% CI 1.60–2.46)
Kim et al. [27]	Retrospective	III	156	62.6 ± 7.1 56.7 ± 13.6	Continuous T-score	T-score was associated with screw loosening following lumbosacral interbody fusion and pedicle screw fixation. T-score was -1.6 ± 1.6 in cases with screw loosening and -0.8 ± 1.5 in cases with screws remaining fixed

Bredow et al. [28]	Retrospective	III	365	59.1 ± 17.2	CT attenuation in HU was used to determine mean bone density of each vertebral body of lumbar and thoracic spine	Decreasing mean CT attenuation was associated with increasing age and increased risk for screw loosening. Bone density was 116.3 ± 53.5 HU in cases with screw loosening and $132.7 \pm 41.$ HU in cases with screws remaining fixed
Liu et al. [29]	Meta-analysis	III	2215	N/A	BMD	In pooled analysis, decreasing BMD was associated with PJK following spinal fusion
Park et al. [30]	Retrospective	III	160	67.6 ± 6.1	Presence of absence of osteoporosis	In adjusted analysis, osteoporosis was independently associated with PJF following ASD surgery
O'Leary et al. [31]	Retrospective	III	44	66 ± 10.3	Continuous T-score used to diagnose osteopenia	Patients with osteopenia had an increased risk of acute fractures when compared to a matched cohort
Yagi et al. [32]	Retrospective	III	157	46.9 (22–81)	Presence of absence of osteoporosis and osteopenia	Patients with osteopenia and osteoporosis had an increase in the incidence of PJK that did not reach significance in ($p = 0.055$)

Our current practice: All patients considered for surgery undergo DEXA screening. Any patient with a T score of less than −1.5 is started on teriparatide 20 ucg SQ daily for 3 months prior to surgery and then 3 months after surgery

Table 7.4 Preoperative – hemoglobin

Author(s)	Study design	Evidence level	N (total)	Mean age, years ± SD; year (range)	Variable evaluated: preoperative hemoglobin	Conclusion
Carabini et al. [33]	Retrospective	III	548	54.9 ± 14.7 (≤4 U transfused) 58.1 ± 15.0 (≥4 U transfused)	Preincision Hb	Preoperative Hb was independently associated with a major transfusion (≥4 U pRBCs) during spine fusion surgery
Lenoir et al. [34]	Retrospective	III	230	61.5 ± 13.6 (transfused) 56.0 ± 17.0 (transfused)	Preoperative Hb	Preoperative Hb level <12 g/dL was independently associated with transfusion during spine surgery (OR 6.7, 95% CI 3.1–17.2)
Nuttall et al. [35]	Retrospective	III	244	47 ± 22	Preoperative Hb	Low (undefined) Hb was associated with increased rate of transfusion
Veeravagu et al. [36]	Retrospective	III	24,774	N/A	Presence of anemia (HCT <36)	In unadjusted analysis, Hct <36 was associated with 1.37-fold increase in wound infection rates.
Zheng et al. [37]	Retrospective	III	112	54 (27–84)	Preoperative Hb and Hct, preoperative anemia	In adjusted analysis, preoperative Hb was independently associated with intraoperative blood loss and transfusion requirements

| Seican et al. [38] | Retrospective | III | 24,473 | 60 ± 15 (severe anemia) 63 ± 13 (moderate anemia) 61 ± 15 (mild anemia) 55 ± 14 (no anemia) | Severe anemia, moderate anemia, mild anemia, no anemia | In a propensity score-matched analysis, all levels of preoperative anemia were associated with increased risk of 30-day complications or increased LOS |

Our current practice: any patient with preoperative Hb level of <12.0 g/dL (female) or <13.5 g/dL (males) is referred to our blood management clinic for a complete diagnostic workup and treatment

Body Mass Index

Obesity is now widely recognized as a significant health problem in the United States and elsewhere. The Centers for Disease Control and Prevention (CDC) currently uses the following ranges and definitions as they relate to body mass index (BMI) status: underweight <18.5 kg/m^2; normal 18.5 kg/m^2 to <25 kg/m^2; overweight 25 kg/m^2 to <30 kg/m^2; obese 30 kg/m^2 or higher. They further categorize obesity as Class 1 (BMI 30 kg/m^2 to <35 kg/m^2), Class 2 (BMI 35 kg/m^2 to <40 kg/m^2), or Class 3 (BMI 40 kg/m^2 or greater).

The literature is replete with studies that identify an association between complications and increasing BMI. The Spine Patient Outcomes Research Trial (SPORT) revealed that obese (BMI $\geq$30 kg/m^2) patients treated for degenerative spondylolisthesis had a higher postoperative infection rate (5% vs. 1%) than nonobese (BMI <30 kg/m^2) patients [39]. Marquez-Lara el al. studied the ASC-NSQIP database and found than wound infection and risk of developing deep-vein thrombosis (DVT) were correlated with increasing BMI [40].

In ASD literature, Soroceanu et al. retrospectively reviewed a multicenter prospective database and found that BMI $\geq$30 kg/m^2 was associated with a higher incidence of major complications and wound infections [41]. Smith et al. found greater BMI was associated with increased risk of rod fracture [42] and Wang et al. found it to be a risk factor for implant failure as well [43]. Bridwell [44] and Park [30] both found that increasing BMI increased the risk of PJK. Yagi et al. [45] however, reported an incidence of PJK of 20% with no difference in the obese and nonobese cohorts.

Our practice has been to counsel our obese patients on the increased risks associated with adult spinal deformity surgery with advancing BMI; and we have established a goal of 35 kg/m^2 for our patients undergoing these rigorous surgeries. We utilize our Weight Management clinic and local hospital dieticians to help our patients with their weight loss. Some ultimately have bariatric surgery to achieve the desired goal but many are able to lose the needed weight through modified eating habits alone (Table 7.5). Improved diabetic control and blood pressure are two of the positive side effects that we have seen with this practice.

Table 7.5 Preoperative – body mass index

Author(s)	Study design	Evidence level	N (total)	Mean age, years ± SD; year (range)	Variable evaluated: body mass index, kg/m²	Conclusion
Rihn et al. [39]	Retrospective	III	1235	N/A	Obese >30 Nonobese ≤30	BMI ˃ 30 kg/m² was associated with higher rate of postoperative infection and reoperation at 4-years follow-up in patients with DS. In patients with SpS, no difference in surgical complications.
Marquez-Lara et al. [40]	Retrospective	III	24,196	56.73 ± 14.9 56.4 ± 16.8	Overweight BMI ≥25 Normal BMI 18.5–24.99	BMI ≥25 kg/m² was associated with increased incidence of DVT, PE, wound infection. BMI ≥40 kg/m² was associated with ARF, sepsis, UTI
Soroceanu et al. [41]	Retrospective	III	241	59.8 ± N/A 53.6 ± N/A	Obese ≥30 Nonobese <30	BMI 30 ≥kg/m² was associated with higher incidence of major complications following ASD surgery. No association with minor complications, radiographic and neurologic complications, and revision surgery

(continued)

Table 7.5 (continued)

Author(s)	Study design	Evidence level	N (total)	Mean age, years ± SD; year (range)	Variable evaluated: body mass index, kg/m²	Conclusion
Smith et al. [42]	Retrospective	IV	287	54.8 ± 15.8	Smoking status obtained from ISSG database	Smoking was not associated with RF following ASD surgery
Wang et al. [43]	Retrospective	III	35	37.4 ± 10.1 37.8 ± 13.3	BMI cut-off 27	BMI >27 kg/m² was associated with instrumentation failure after pVCR in ASD patients
Bridwell et al. [44]	Retrospective	III	90	49.9 ± 12.6	Continuous BMI values grouped by PJK status	Increase in BMI was associated with higher incidence of PJK following ASD surgery
Park et al. [30]	Retrospective	III	160	67.6 ± 6.1	Presence of absence of osteoporosis	In adjusted analysis, osteoporosis was independently associated with PJF following ASD surgery
Yagi et al. [45]	Retrospective	III	157	46.9 (22–81)	Presence of absence of osteoporosis and osteopenia diagnosed using T-score and WHO criteria	Patients with osteopenia and osteoporosis had an increase in the incidence of PJK that did not reach signifance in ($p = 0.055$)

Our current practice: patients with BMI greater than 35 kg/m² are referred to our weight management clinic

Frailty

Frailty is defined as age-associated declines in physiologic reserves and function across several organ systems. The modified Frailty Index (mFI), a scale that uses 11 of the 70 variables proposed by the Canadian Study of Health and Aging Frailty Index (CSHA-FI), has been studied in its association with increased complications and reoperations in patients undergoing spine surgery. Four studies have been identified using the mFI; they showed increasing complications with increasing levels of frailty [46–49] (Table 7.6).

We believe this is an important part of the preoperative patient assessment prior to major spinal deformity surgery; however, whether this is modifiable or not remains a controversial topic. We are not aware of any peer-reviewed studies that have shown either the modifiability of a frail individual or if this modification resets their risk to that of a non-frail individual. The idea of "prehabilitation" of patients prior to surgery is appealing and is currently the subject of a prospective study at one major spine center.

Hemoglobin A1c

Diabetes Mellitus is currently an epidemic in the United States and parts of Europe and is a leading cause of death and disability in the Western world. Hemoglobin A1c (HbA1c) is a glycated hemoglobin used to measure the average amount of glucose in the blood over the previous 2–3 months. A normal level is below 5.7%; prediabetes is an HbA1c level between 5.7% and 6.4%; and diabetes is generally identified as an HbA1c level of 6.5% or higher.

It has been postulated that risk factors associated with surgery in diabetics are not weighted equally and that improved diabetic control can lessen the risk of complications with surgery. We have identified three papers in the literature that tested for an association between complications after spine surgery and increasing HbA1c levels. Walid et al. [50] evaluated 122 patients and found increasing cost associated with increasing HbA1c. Takahashi et al. [51] found higher rates of non-union for patients with HbA1c levels

Table 7.6 Preoperative – frailty

Author(s)	Study design	Evidence level	N (total)	Mean age, years ± SD	Variable evaluated: frailty	Conclusion
Shin et al. [46]	Retrospective	III	6965	ACDF group: 52.9 ± N/A PCF group: 59.8 ± N/A	mFI	Frailty severity was an independent predictor of complications in patients undergoing cervical fusion.
Leven et al. [47]	Retrospective	III	1001	59.2 ± 14.8	mFI	Frailty severity was an independent predictor of postoperative complications, mortality, and return to the operating room.
Flexman et al. [48]	Retrospective	III	53,080	56.1 ± 14.5	mFI	Frailty severity was an independent predictor of worsened postoperative outcomes.
Ali et al. [49]	Retrospective	III	18,294	N/A	mFI	Increasing mFI score was associated with a higher risk of postoperative morbidity and mortality.

Our current practice does not include an assessment of frailty exceeding 6.5%. A final study by Hikata et al. [52] found that diabetic patients who developed a surgical site infection after surgery had increased HbA1c levels at the time of reoperation for the infection compared to prior to surgery.

Measuring HbA1c level is part of our standard work in patients being considered for ASD surgery; we established an HbA1c level cutoff of 7%. Any patient with an elevated HbA1c level is referred back to their primary care physician or to our diabetes clinic for tighter management prior to surgery (Table 7.7).

Mental Health

Impaired mental health has been known for years to affect spinal complaints [53]. Despite this knowledge, exactly how to evaluate and then treat this cohort of patients has been not been universally established. The literature reflects this – our review of existing studies found thirteen that showed a correlation between impaired mental health and diminished outcomes after spine surgery; however, there was tremendous variability in the measures used to evaluate mental health. Most commonly, the Zung Depression Scale (ZDS) has been used to measure depression. Studies using ZDS have demonstrated worse improvement after surgery [54–58] with increasing ZDS scores. Similarly, the mental health component (MCS) of the Short Form-36 (SF-36) [59] has been found to be predictive of decreased improvement after surgery [60, 61]. Although some have shown that despite low MCS, patients can still demonstrate improvement after surgery [62, 63]. Lastly, Urban-Baeza et al. used the Beck Depression Inventory to evaluate patients undergoing spinal stenosis surgery. In this study, those with depressive symptoms had worse outcomes at 1 year [64]. All of these reports highlight the varied approaches spine surgeons are using to evaluate their patients prior to surgery.

We made the SRS-22r [65] part of our standard work in the clinic. The Mental Health Domain of the SRS-22r questionnaire was adapted with permission from the MCS portion of the SF-36. We utilize this as our screening tool for depressive symptoms. Any patient with a domain score under 2.5 is evaluated for the need for mental health referral, though it is rare for any patient to have their surgery delayed because of this (Table 7.8).

Table 7.7 Preoperative – hemoglobin A1c

Author(s)	Study design	Evidence level	N (total)	Mean age, years ± SD	Variable evaluated: hemoglobin A1c	Conclusion
Walid et al. [50]	Retrospective	III	442	LMD no DM: 60 ± 14 LMD HbA1C: 59 ± 11 LMD DM: 69 ± 9 ACDF no DM: 52 ± 10 ACDF HbA1c: 58 ± 9 ACDF DM: 60 ± 10 LDF no DM: 55 ± 13 LDF HbA1c: 54 ± 10 LDF DM: 59 ± 7	History of DM; HbA1c screening cutpoint 6.1%	When adjusted for age, BMI, or both, preoperative HbA1c value and DM status were not associated with increased LOS and cost.

Takahashi et al. [51]	Retrospective	III	165	DM group: 70.9 ± 7.2 Non-DM group: 68.6 ± 8.1	Diabetes diagnosis, HbA1c (<6.5% or ≥6.5%), disease duration, insulin use	Patients with a history of DM (>20 years) or Hb1c level greater than 6.5% were less likely to have improvement in low back pain. Patients with a history of DM (>20 years) or insulin use were less likely to have improvement in leg numbness.
Hikata et al. [52]	Retrospective	III	345	DM group: 64.3 ± N/A Non-DM group: 63.8 ± N/A	Preoperative HbA1c (%) values	Patients who developed SSI had a higher mean HbA1c (%) value than the cohort without surgical site infection (7.6 vs. 6.9, p 0.006).

Our current practice: any patient with a preoperative HbA1c level greater than 7% is referred to their primary care physician or to our diabetes clinic for tighter management prior to surgery

Table 7.8 Preoperative – mental health

Author(s)	Study design	Evidence level	N (total)	Mean age, years ± SD	Variable evaluated: mental health	Conclusion
Waddel et al. [53]	Case-control	II	320	N/A	Eysenck Personality, MSPQ, ZDS, Sternback Health Index, Pilowsky Illness Behavior	Psychological or behavioral factors were not "causative" of the physical problem. Subjective disability correlated with physical, psychologic, and behavioral factors; with little influence noted from social or demographic factors.
Hägg et al. [54]	RCT	II	264	Surgical group improved: 43 ± 8.8 Surgical group with no improvement: 42 ± 7.3 Non-surgical group improved: 41 ± 6.8 Non-surgical group with no improvement: 45 ± 7.7	KSP, SCID II questionnaire, ZDS	Preoperative depressive symptoms were predictive of functional outcomes in the non-surgical cohort.

Chaichana et al. [55]	Prospective cohort	III	67	41 ± 10	ZDS; MSPQ	Preoperative depression and somatic anxiety were associated with decreased likelihood of reaching an MCID in disability.
Adogwa et al. [56]	Retrospective	III	69	70 ± 4.50	ZDS	Increasing Zung score was associated with decreased improvement following revision lumbar surgery.
Adogwa et al. [57]	Retrospective	III	53	56.27 ± 12.48	ZDS	Increasing Zung score was predictive of patient dissatisfaction following revision lumbar surgery.
Adogwa et al. [58]	Retrospective	III	150	57 ± 11	ZDS	After adjusting for age, BMI, disease/symptom duration, smoking, comorbidities and level of preoperative pain and disability, increasing Zung score was associated with decreased improvement in disability.
Ware et al. [59]	Case-control	II	379	N/A	Health status, 9-item questionnaire	Patient data used to develop the MOS SF-36 was shown in this report.

(continued)

Table 7.8 (continued)

Author(s)	Study design	Evidence level	N (total)	Mean age, years ± SD	Variable evaluated: mental health	Conclusion
Trief et al. [60]	Retrospective	III	160	44.22 ± 8.59	MCS	Lower preoperative MCS values were associated with increased postoperative pain and worse physical function after surgery.
Carr et al. [61]	Cohort	III	79	No postop pain group: 47.8 ± N/A Postop pain group: 48.9 ± N/A	MCS	Increase in SF-36 MCS values was correlated with significantly lower postoperative neck pain ($p = 0.003$) and NDI scores ($p = 0.004$).
Baksheshian et al. [62]	Retrospective	III	144	LMH group: 59.3 ± 9.6 HMH group: 52.8 ± 18.3	MCS	LMH cohort (≤25th percentile MCS score) was less likely to reach an MCID on the PCS ($p < 0.05$) after adjusting for covariates.
Theis et al. [63]	Systematic review	IV	188	38 ± N/A	SF-36	Fair quality data demonstrating HRQoL improvement following surgery.
Urban-Baeza et al. [64]	Cohort	III	58	Depressed: $57^{\bar{x}} \pm 11$ Nondepressed: $56^{\bar{x}} \pm 10$	Beck depression inventory	Decrease in depressive symptoms 1 year following surgery for spinal stenosis ($p = 0.001$).

| Asher et al. [65] | Prospective observational case series | III | 111 | 27.2 ± 16.3 | Refined SRS-22 HRQoL | Internal consistency of the SRS-22 function domain was improved following slight modifications to question 18; and slightly decreased after removal of question 15. |

Our current practice: SRS-22r is used as a screening tool for depressive symptoms. Any patient with a domain score under 2.5 is further evaluated for a mental health referral, though it is rare for any patient to have their surgery significantly delayed

Vitamin D

Vitamin D is produced by the body in response to exposure of the skin to sunlight. It also occurs naturally in some foods such as fish, egg yolk, and fortified dairy. Vitamin D is essential for the body to utilize calcium for proper mineralization of bone. The two commonly measured forms of Vitamin D are Vitamin D2 (ergo-calciferol) and Vitamin D3 (cholecalciferol). Both of these can be converted in the body into 25-hydroxyvitamin D (25(OH)D) and 1,25-dihydroxyvitamin D (1,25(OH)2D), the inactive and active forms of the vitamin respectively.

Early reports linked low levels of Vitamin D to increased complications [66–68] (Table 7.9). More recent investigations evaluating the stable form of the vitamin also found that pseudoarthrosis was associated with diminished vitamin levels [66, 67]. Since an older study found no difference between low levels of 1,25-(OH)2D and pseudoarthrosis [68], more research is needed in this area.

We currently measure 25(OH)D levels in all patients. Our protocol for supplementation sets a goal of 30 ng/ml for 25(OH)D. If patient's level is 20–30 ng/ml, we supplement with 1000 units/day of Vitamin D3. A level of 10–20 ng/ml receives 2000 units/day (above anything they may be taking). If they start below 20 ng/ml, we usually recheck in 3–6 months, though we do not delay their surgery for this. If the deficiency is severe, <10 ng/ml, we typically refer to our bone health clinic to evaluate them for malabsorption syndromes.

Intraoperative Factors

Fluid Management

A goal-directed fluid therapy (GDFT) approach is one in which the surgical team preoperatively plans perioperative hemodynamic management to optimize outcomes. There remains considerable debate about the merits of the type of fluid used in the perioperative period (colloid vs. crystalloid), the total volume delivered (liberal vs. restrictive), whether there should exist specific goals driving the administration of fluid (goal-directed vs. not goal-directed). We evaluated the literature and found moderate evidence

Table 7.9 Preoperative – vitamin D

Author(s)	Study design	evidence level	N (total)	Mean age, years ± SD	Variable evaluated: vitamin d	Conclusion
Kerezoudis et al. [66]	Systematic review	II	264	Variable	Variable cutoff value	Preoperative vitamin D deficiency may be associated with lower fusion rates and recurrent-persistent low back pain.
Ravindra et al. [67]	Cohort	III	133	57.6 ± 12.7	25(OH)D levels <20 ng/mL	Both nonunion at 12 months and time to fusion were increased in the cohort with vitamin D deficiency. When adjusted for confounding variables, vitamin D deficiency was independently associated with nonunion (OR 3.449, $p = 0.045$).
Schofferman et al. [68]	Retrospective	III	47	41	Not stated for 1,25-[OH]2 D3 form evaluated in the publication.	Vitamin D deficiency was not correlated with pseudoarthrosis.

Our current practice: We currently measure 25(OH)D levels in all patients. Our protocol for supplementation sets a goal of 30 ng/mL for 25(OH)D. If patient's level is 20–30 ng/mL, we supplement with 1000 units/day of Vitamin D3. A level of 10–20 ng/mL receives 2000 units/day (above anything they may be taking). If they start below 20 ng/mL, we usually recheck in 3–6 months, though we do not delay their surgery for this. If the deficiency is severe, <10 ng/ml, we typically refer to our bone health clinic to evaluate them for malabsorption syndromes that a goal-directed fluid therapy strategy produces better results [7, 69–76] (Table 7.10).

Corcoran et al. [69] performed a meta-analysis and found that patients who were managed with GDFT had reduced risk of pneumonia, renal complications, pulmonary edema, and had a shorter length of stay compared to liberal fluid therapy (LFT) cohort. Gan et al. [70] performed a prospective, randomized controlled trial (RCT) comparing the use of an algorithmic approach to fluid management using real-time measurement of stroke volume to customary treatment. They found the control group had longer length of stay, more nausea and vomiting, and tolerated a regular diet later than the experimental group. In a similar study, Scheeren et al. [71] found GDFT use led to decreased wound infection.

Peng et al. [73] performed an RCT comparing GDFT to LFT in patients undergoing orthopedic surgery and found that GDFT had fewer hypotensive episodes, less intraoperative volume given, and shorter time to flatus. Bacchin et al. [75] found similar results when analyzing this method in spine surgery patients.

Implementation of this approach is more difficult than modifying patient's parameters as it requires the cooperation of our anesthesia colleagues. The evidence for it, primarily found in the anesthesia literature, is compelling. We have found that approaching our anesthesia department in a collaborative and evidence-based manner has been well received and we are currently implementing this approach for our spinal deformity surgeries.

Tranexamic Acid

Tranexamic acid (TXA) is a synthetic derivative of the amino acid lysine. It reversibly blocks the lysine binding sites on plasminogen molecules inhibiting the interaction of plasminogen with fibrin and preventing the dissolution of the fibrin clot. Consequently, TXA decreases blood loss, minimizes the need for allogeneic blood transfusions, and prevents clotting abnormalities after surgery. This hemostatic agent is commonly used in spinal deformity surgery and has been extensively investigated in recent years. We identified three meta-analyses of RCTs that support its use [77–79] (Table 7.11).

Table 7.10 Intraoperative – fluid management

Author(s)	Study design	Evidence level	N (total)	Mean age, years ± SD	Variable evaluated: fluid management (FM)	Conclusion
Sethi et al. [7]	Retrospective	III	164	Group A: 62; Group B: 64	Modified anesthesia protocol	Significant reduction in perioperative complication rates (16% vs. 52%, $p < 0.001$) in group that received modified anesthesia protocol.
Corcoran et al. [69]	Systematic review	I	5021	Variable	LFT and GDFT	GDFT use resulted in improved outcomes when compared to a liberal approach. GD not compared to restrictive.
Gan et al. [70]	RCT	II	100	Control: 59 ± 12 Protocol: 56 ± 13	GDFT	GDFT cohort had improved postoperative outcomes.
Scheeren et al. [71]	RCT	II	52	Control: 73 ± 9 Protocol: 68 ± 9	GDFT	GDFT led to reduction in postoperative wound infections ($p < 0.01$).
Hamilton et al. [72]	Systematic Review & Meta-Analysis	I	4805	Variable	Perioperative hemodynamic interventions:	Meta-analysis of 23 studies reporting the number of complications showed that preemptive hemodynamic interventions led to a reduction in overall complications (OR 0.43 [0.34–0.53].

(continued)

Table 7.10 (continued)

Author(s)	Study design	Evidence level	N (total)	Mean age, years ± SD	Variable evaluated: fluid management (FM)	Conclusion
Peng et al. [73]	RCT	II	80	Control: 53 ± 10 Protocol: 55 ± 13	GDFT	No differences in LOS, complications or mortality. GD cohort with reduced incidence of hypotensive events ($p < 0.05$), less transfusion requirements ($p < 0.05$).
Brienza et al. [74]	Meta-analysis	I	4220	Variable	Hemodynamic optimization	Hemodynamic optimization reduced incidence of renal dysfunction and mortality ($p = 0.004$).
Bacchin et al. [75]	Retrospective	III	45	LFT group:22 ± 3.4; GDFT group: 23 ± 5.2	GDFT	GDFT cohort had reduced transfusion requirements and improved postoperative outcomes.
Glance et al. [76]	Retrospective	III	10,100	Not transfused: 60.2 ± N/A Transfused: 64.6 ± N/A	Intraoperative transfusion	Intraoperative blood transfusion was associated with higher mortality and postoperative complications.

Our current practice: implementation of this approach is more difficult than modifying patient's parameters as it requires the cooperation of our anesthesia colleagues. The evidence for it, primarily found in the anesthesia literature, is compelling. We have found that approaching our anesthesia department in a collaborative and evidence-based manner has been well received, and we are currently implementing this approach for our spinal deformity surgeries

Table 7.11 Intraoperative – tranexamic acid

Author(s)	Study design	Evidence level	N (total)	Mean age, years ± SD	Variable evaluated: TXA	Conclusion
Yan et al.	Meta-analysis	I	482	Variable	IV TXA IV EACA	Patients who received TXA had reduction in blood loss ($p = 0.01$), reduced blood transfusion ($p = 0.008$), reduced blood transfusion rate ($p = 0.01$). There was no significant difference in the incidence of DVT between the two groups.
Zhang et al.	Meta-analysis	I	411	Variable	Six protocols describing IV TXA use. Placebo group in all included RCTs.	Patients who received TXA had reduction in blood loss, blood transfusion requirements, and postoperative PTT with weighted MD of −1.59 [95% CI: −3.07, −0.10].
Cheriyan et al.	Meta-analysis	I	644	Variable	Variable IV TXA protocols	Intraoperative, postoperative, and total blood loss significantly reduced in the TXA cohort ($p < 0.05$). Blood transfusion requirements higher in the placebo group ($p < 0.05$).

Our current practice: The question remains as to the best dose for TXA. Currently the most common dosages vary from 10 mg/kg loading dose and 1 mg/kg/h maintenance during surgery (low dose protocol) to 100 mg/kg loading dose and 10 mg/kg/h maintenance infusion (high dose protocol). Others have used various dosages in between. Which of these is most efficacious and safe is not clear, though several studies are currently ongoing. In our practice, we have used the lose dose protocol for the past 3 years. Since implementation, we have not had to transfuse with platelets or fresh frozen plasma (FFP) in our patients undergoing major adult spinal deformity surgery, including several with pedicle subtraction osteotomies

Yuan, et al. [77] pooled data from six placebo-controlled RCTs ($n = 411$) and found a reduction in blood loss and need for transfusion in the TXA group. Zhang et al. [78] found similar results in another meta-analysis. Cheriyan et al. [79] combined the findings of eleven RCTs ($n = 644$) undergoing spine surgery and found less blood loss and lower transfusions in the TXA group.

The question remains as to the best dose for TXA. Currently the most common dosages vary from 10 mg/kg loading dose and 1 mg/kg/h maintenance during surgery (low dose protocol) to 100 mg/kg loading dose and 10 mg/kg/h maintenance infusion (high dose protocol). Others have used various dosages in between. Which of these is most efficacious and safe is not clear, though several studies are currently ongoing. In our practice, we have used the lose dose protocol for the past 3 years. Since implementation, we have not had to transfuse with platelets or fresh frozen plasma (FFP) in our patients undergoing major adult spinal deformity surgery, including several with pedicle subtraction osteotomies.

Conclusion

Our surgical techniques and implants to treat adult spinal deformity have progressed remarkably over the last 20 years; however, our complication rates remain unacceptably high. Standardizing the optimization of patients' co-morbidities and intraoperative management has the potential to help us reduce these complications and enable us to deliver better and safer care for the growing number of patients with adult spinal deformity.

References

1. Schwab F, Dubey A, Gamez L, El Fegoun AB, Hwang K, Pagala M, et al. Adult scoliosis: prevalence, SF-36, and nutritional parameters in an elderly volunteer population. Spine. 2005;30(9):1082–5.
2. Diebo BG, Lafage V, Varghese JJ, Gupta M, Kim HJ, Ames C, et al. After 9 years of 3-column osteotomies, are we doing better? Performance curve analysis of 573 surgeries with 2-year follow-up. Neurosurgery. 2018;83(1):69–75.

3. Smith JS, Lafage V, Shaffrey CI, Schwab F, Lafage R, Hostin R, et al. Outcomes of operative and nonoperative treatment for adult spinal deformity: a prospective, multicenter, propensity-matched cohort assessment with minimum 2-year follow-up. Neurosurgery. 2016;78(6):851–61.
4. Smith JS, Klineberg E, Lafage V, Shaffrey CI, Schwab F, Lafage R, et al. Prospective multicenter assessment of perioperative and minimum 2-year postoperative complication rates associated with adult spinal deformity surgery. J Neurosurg Spine. 2016;25(1):1–14.
5. McCarthy I, O'Brien M, Ames C, Robinson C, Errico T, Polly DW Jr, et al. Incremental cost-effectiveness of adult spinal deformity surgery: observed quality-adjusted life years with surgery compared with predicted quality-adjusted life years without surgery. Neurosurg Focus. 2014;36(5):E3.
6. Halpin RJ, Sugrue PA, Gould RW, Kallas PG, Schafer MF, Ondra SL, et al. Standardizing care for high-risk patients in spine surgery: the Northwestern high-risk spine protocol. Spine. 2010;35(25):2232–8.
7. Sethi RK, Pong RP, Leveque JC, Dean TC, Olivar SJ, Rupp SM. The Seattle spine team approach to adult deformity surgery: a systems-based approach to perioperative care and subsequent reduction in perioperative complication rates. Spine Deform. 2014;2(2):95–103.
8. Black JR, Miller D. The Toyota way to healthcare excellence: increase efficiency and improve quality with Lean. Chicago: Health Administration Press; 2008. xiii, 255 p.
9. Schoenfeld AJ, Carey PA, Cleveland AW 3rd, Bader JO, Bono CM. Patient factors, comorbidities, and surgical characteristics that increase mortality and complication risk after spinal arthrodesis: a prognostic study based on 5,887 patients. Spine J. 2013;13(10):1171–9.
10. Adogwa O, Elsamadicy AA, Mehta AI, Cheng J, Bagley CA, Karikari IO. Preoperative nutritional status is an independent predictor of 30-day hospital readmission after elective spine surgery. Spine. 2016;41(17):1400–4.
11. Adogwa O, Martin JR, Huang K, Verla T, Fatemi P, Thompson P, et al. Preoperative serum albumin level as a predictor of postoperative complication after spine fusion. Spine. 2014;39(18):1513–9.
12. Tempel Z, Grandhi R, Maserati M, Panczykowski D, Ochoa J, Russavage J, et al. Prealbumin as a serum biomarker of impaired perioperative nutritional status and risk for surgical site infection after spine surgery. J Neurol Surg A Cent Eur Neurosurg. 2015;76(2):139–43.
13. Bohl DD, Shen MR, Mayo BC, Massel DH, Long WW, Modi KD, et al. Malnutrition predicts infectious and wound complications following posterior lumbar spinal fusion. Spine. 2016;41(21):1693–9.
14. Fu MC, Buerba RA, Grauer JN. Preoperative nutritional status as an adjunct predictor of major postoperative complications following anterior cervical discectomy and fusion. Clin Spine Surg. 2016;29(4):167–72.
15. Freedman ND, Leitzmann MF, Hollenbeck AR, Schatzkin A, Abnet CC. Cigarette smoking and subsequent risk of lung cancer in men and women: analysis of a prospective cohort study. Lancet Oncol. 2008;9(7):649–56.

16. Freedman ND, Silverman DT, Hollenbeck AR, Schatzkin A, Abnet CC. Association between smoking and risk of bladder cancer among men and women. JAMA. 2011;306(7):737–45.

17. Tang H, Zhu J, Ji F, Wang S, Xie Y, Fei H. Risk factors for postoperative complication after spinal fusion and instrumentation in degenerative lumbar scoliosis patients. J Orthop Surg Res. 2014;9(1):15.

18. Soroceanu A, Burton DC, Oren JH, Smith JS, Hostin R, Shaffrey CI, et al. Medical complications after adult spinal deformity surgery: incidence, risk factors, and clinical impact. Spine. 2016;41(22):1718–23.

19. Martin CT, Gao Y, Duchman KR, Pugely AJ. The impact of current smoking and smoking cessation on short-term morbidity risk after lumbar spine surgery. Spine. 2016;41(7):577–84.

20. McCunniff PT, Young ES, Ahmadinia K, Ahn UM, Ahn NU. Smoking is associated with increased blood loss and transfusion use after lumbar spinal surgery. Clin Orthop Relat Res. 2016;474(4):1019–25.

21. Inoue S, Khashan M, Fujimori T, Berven SH. Analysis of mechanical failure associated with reoperation in spinal fusion to the sacrum in adult spinal deformity. J Orthop Sci. 2015;20(4):609–16.

22. Mok JM, Cloyd JM, Bradford DS, Hu SS, Deviren V, Smith JA, et al. Reoperation after primary fusion for adult spinal deformity: rate, reason, and timing. Spine. 2009;34(8):832–9.

23. Puvanesarajah V, Shen FH, Cancienne JM, Novicoff WM, Jain A, Shimer AL, et al. Risk factors for revision surgery following primary adult spinal deformity surgery in patients 65 years and older. J Neurosurg Spine. 2016;25(4):486–93.

24. Carlson BB, Burton DC, Jackson RS, Robinson S. Recidivism rates after smoking cessation before spinal fusion. Orthopedics. 2016;39(2):e318–22.

25. Hymowitz N, Cummings KM, Hyland A, Lynn WR, Pechacek TF, Hartwell TD. Predictors of smoking cessation in a cohort of adult smokers followed for five years. Tob Control. 1997;6(Suppl 2):S57–62.

26. Okuyama K, Abe E, Suzuki T, Tamura Y, Chiba M, Sato K. Influence of bone mineral density on pedicle screw fixation: a study of pedicle screw fixation augmenting posterior lumbar interbody fusion in elderly patients. Spine J. 2001;1(6):402–7.

27. Kim JB, Park SW, Lee YS, Nam TK, Park YS, Kim YB. The effects of spinopelvic parameters and paraspinal muscle degeneration on S1 screw loosening. J Korean Neurosurg Soc. 2015;58(4):357–62.

28. Bredow J, Boese CK, Werner CM, Siewe J, Lohrer L, Zarghooni K, et al. Predictive validity of preoperative CT scans and the risk of pedicle screw loosening in spinal surgery. Arch Orthop Trauma Surg. 2016;136(8):1063–7.

29. Liu FY, Wang T, Yang SD, Wang H, Yang DL, Ding WY. Incidence and risk factors for proximal junctional kyphosis: a meta-analysis. Eur Spine J. 2016;25(8):2376–83.

30. Park SJ, Lee CS, Chung SS, Lee JY, Kang SS, Park SH. Different risk factors of proximal junctional kyphosis and proximal junctional failure

following long instrumented fusion to the sacrum for adult spinal deformity: survivorship analysis of 160 patients. Neurosurgery. 2017;80(2):279–86.

31. O'Leary PT, Bridwell KH, Lenke LG, Good CR, Pichelmann MA, Buchowski JM, et al. Risk factors and outcomes for catastrophic failures at the top of long pedicle screw constructs: a matched cohort analysis performed at a single center. Spine. 2009;34(20):2134–9.

32. Yagi M, Ohne H, Konomi T, Fujiyoshi K, Kaneko S, Komiyama T, et al. Teriparatide improves volumetric bone mineral density and fine bone structure in the UIV+1 vertebra, and reduces bone failure type PJK after surgery for adult spinal deformity. Osteoporos Int. 2016;27(12):3495–502.

33. Carabini LM, Zeeni C, Moreland NC, Gould RW, Avram MJ, Hemmer LB, et al. Development and validation of a generalizable model for predicting major transfusion during spine fusion surgery. J Neurosurg Anesthesiol. 2014;26(3):205–15.

34. Lenoir B, Merckx P, Paugam-Burtz C, Dauzac C, Agostini MM, Guigui P, et al. Individual probability of allogeneic erythrocyte transfusion in elective spine surgery: the predictive model of transfusion in spine surgery. Anesthesiology. 2009;110(5):1050–60.

35. Nuttall GA, Horlocker TT, Santrach PJ, Oliver WC Jr, Dekutoski MB, Bryant S. Predictors of blood transfusions in spinal instrumentation and fusion surgery. Spine. 2000;25(5):596–601.

36. Veeravagu A, Patil CG, Lad SP, Boakye M. Risk factors for postoperative spinal wound infections after spinal decompression and fusion surgeries. Spine. 2009;34(17):1869–72.

37. Zheng F, Cammisa FP Jr, Sandhu HS, Girardi FP, Khan SN. Factors predicting hospital stay, operative time, blood loss, and transfusion in patients undergoing revision posterior lumbar spine decompression, fusion, and segmental instrumentation. Spine. 2002;27(8):818–24.

38. Seicean A, Seicean S, Alan N, Schiltz NK, Rosenbaum BP, Jones PK, et al. Preoperative anemia and perioperative outcomes in patients who undergo elective spine surgery. Spine. 2013;38(15):1331–41.

39. Rihn JA, Radcliff K, Hilibrand AS, Anderson DT, Zhao W, Lurie J, et al. Does obesity affect outcomes of treatment for lumbar stenosis and degenerative spondylolisthesis? Analysis of the Spine Patient Outcomes Research Trial (SPORT). Spine. 2012;37(23):1933–46.

40. Marquez-Lara A, Nandyala SV, Sankaranarayanan S, Noureldin M, Singh K. Body mass index as a predictor of complications and mortality after lumbar spine surgery. Spine. 2014;39(10):798–804.

41. Soroceanu A, Burton DC, Diebo BG, Smith JS, Hostin R, Shaffrey CI, et al. Impact of obesity on complications, infection, and patient-reported outcomes in adult spinal deformity surgery. J Neurosurg Spine. 2015;23:1–9.

42. Smith JS, Shaffrey E, Klineberg E, Shaffrey CI, Lafage V, Schwab FJ, et al. Prospective multicenter assessment of risk factors for rod fracture

following surgery for adult spinal deformity. J Neurosurg Spine. 2014;21(6):994–1003.

43. Wang H, Guo J, Wang S, Yang Y, Zhang Y, Qiu G, et al. Instrumentation failure after posterior vertebral column resection in adult spinal deformity. Spine. 2017;42(7):471–8.

44. Bridwell KH, Lenke LG, Cho SK, Pahys JM, Zebala LP, Dorward IG, et al. Proximal junctional kyphosis in primary adult deformity surgery: evaluation of 20 degrees as a critical angle. Neurosurgery. 2013;72(6):899–906.

45. Yagi M, Akilah KB, Boachie-Adjei O. Incidence, risk factors and classification of proximal junctional kyphosis: surgical outcomes review of adult idiopathic scoliosis. Spine. 2011;36(1):E60–8.

46. Shin JI, Kothari P, Phan K, Kim JS, Leven D, Lee NJ, et al. Frailty index as a predictor of adverse postoperative outcomes in patients undergoing cervical spinal fusion. Spine. 2017;42(5):304–10.

47. Leven DM, Lee NJ, Kothari P, Steinberger J, Guzman J, Skovrlj B, et al. Frailty index is a significant predictor of complications and mortality after surgery for adult spinal deformity. Spine. 2016;41(23):E1394–E401.

48. Flexman AM, Charest-Morin R, Stobart L, Street J, Ryerson CJ. Frailty and postoperative outcomes in patients undergoing surgery for degenerative spine disease. Spine J. 2016;16(11):1315–23.

49. Ali R, Schwalb JM, Nerenz DR, Antoine HJ, Rubinfeld I. Use of the modified frailty index to predict 30-day morbidity and mortality from spine surgery. J Neurosurg Spine. 2016;25(4):537–41.

50. Walid MS, Newman BF, Yelverton JC, Nutter JP, Ajjan M, Robinson JS Jr. Prevalence of previously unknown elevation of glycosylated hemoglobin in spine surgery patients and impact on length of stay and total cost. J Hosp Med. 2010;5(1):E10–4.

51. Takahashi S, Suzuki A, Toyoda H, Terai H, Dohzono S, Yamada K, et al. Characteristics of diabetes associated with poor improvements in clinical outcomes after lumbar spine surgery. Spine. 2013;38(6):516–22.

52. Hikata T, Iwanami A, Hosogane N, Watanabe K, Ishii K, Nakamura M, et al. High preoperative hemoglobin A1c is a risk factor for surgical site infection after posterior thoracic and lumbar spinal instrumentation surgery. J Orthop Sci. 2014;19(2):223–8.

53. Waddell G, Main CJ, Morris EW, Di Paola M, Gray IC. Chronic low-back pain, psychologic distress, and illness behavior. Spine. 1984;9(2):209–13.

54. Hagg O, Fritzell P, Ekselius L, Nordwall A, Swedish Lumbar Spine Study. Predictors of outcome in fusion surgery for chronic low back pain. A report from the Swedish Lumbar Spine Study. Eur Spine J. 2003;12(1):22–33.

55. Chaichana KL, Mukherjee D, Adogwa O, Cheng JS, McGirt MJ. Correlation of preoperative depression and somatic perception scales with postoperative disability and quality of life after lumbar discectomy. J Neurosurg Spine. 2011;14(2):261–7.

56. Adogwa O, Verla T, Thompson P, Penumaka A, Kudyba K, Johnson K, et al. Affective disorders influence clinical outcomes after revision lumbar surgery in elderly patients with symptomatic adjacent-segment disease, recurrent stenosis, or pseudarthrosis: clinical article. J Neurosurg Spine. 2014;21(2):153–9.

57. Adogwa O, Parker SL, Shau DN, Mendenhall SK, Bydon A, Cheng JS, et al. Preoperative Zung depression scale predicts patient satisfaction independent of the extent of improvement after revision lumbar surgery. Spine J. 2013;13(5):501–6.

58. Adogwa O, Parker SL, Shau DN, Mendenhall SK, Aaronson OS, Cheng JS, et al. Preoperative Zung Depression Scale predicts outcome after revision lumbar surgery for adjacent segment disease, recurrent stenosis, and pseudarthrosis. Spine J. 2012;12(3):179–85.

59. Ware JE Jr, Sherbourne CD. The MOS 36-item short-form health survey (SF-36). I. Conceptual framework and item selection. Med Care. 1992;30(6):473–83.

60. Trief PM, Ploutz-Snyder R, Fredrickson BE. Emotional health predicts pain and function after fusion: a prospective multicenter study. Spine. 2006;31(7):823–30.

61. Carr FA, Healy KM, Villavicencio AT, Nelson EL, Mason A, Burneikiene S, et al. Effect on clinical outcomes of patient pain expectancies and preoperative mental component summary scores from the 36-item short form health survey following anterior cervical discectomy and fusion. J Neurosurg Spine. 2011;15(5):486–90.

62. Bakhsheshian J, Scheer JK, Gum JL, Hostin R, Lafage V, Bess S, et al. Impact of poor mental health in adult spinal deformity patients with poor physical function: a retrospective analysis with a 2-year follow-up. J Neurosurg Spine. 2017;26(1):116–24.

63. Theis J, Gerdhem P, Abbott A. Quality of life outcomes in surgically treated adult scoliosis patients: a systematic review. Eur Spine J. 2015;24(7):1343–55.

64. Urban-Baeza A, Zarate-Kalfopulos B, Romero-Vargas S, Obil-Chavarria C, Brenes-Rojas L, Reyes-Sanchez A. Influence of depression symptoms on patient expectations and clinical outcomes in the surgical management of spinal stenosis. J Neurosurg Spine. 2015;22(1):75–9.

65. Asher MA, Lai SM, Glattes RC, Burton DC, Alanay A, Bago J. Refinement of the SRS-22 health-related quality of life questionnaire function domain. Spine. 2006;31(5):593–7.

66. Kerezoudis P, Rinaldo L, Drazin D, Kallmes D, Krauss W, Hassoon A, et al. Association between vitamin D deficiency and outcomes following spinal fusion surgery: a systematic review. World Neurosurg. 2016;95:71–6.

67. Ravindra VM, Godzik J, Dailey AT, Schmidt MH, Bisson EF, Hood RS, et al. Vitamin D levels and 1-year fusion outcomes in elective spine surgery: a prospective observational study. Spine. 2015;40(19):1536–41.

68. Schofferman J, Schofferman L, Zucherman J, Hsu K, White A. Metabolic bone disease in lumbar pseudarthrosis. Spine. 1990;15(7):687–9.
69. Corcoran T, Rhodes JE, Clarke S, Myles PS, Ho KM. Perioperative fluid management strategies in major surgery: a stratified meta-analysis. Anesth Analg. 2012;114(3):640–51.
70. Gan TJ, Soppitt A, Maroof M, el-Moalem H, Robertson KM, Moretti E, et al. Goal-directed intraoperative fluid administration reduces length of hospital stay after major surgery. Anesthesiology. 2002;97(4):820–6.
71. Scheeren TW, Wiesenack C, Gerlach H, Marx G. Goal-directed intraoperative fluid therapy guided by stroke volume and its variation in high-risk surgical patients: a prospective randomized multicentre study. J Clin Monit Comput. 2013;27(3):225–33.
72. Hamilton MA, Cecconi M, Rhodes A. A systematic review and meta-analysis on the use of preemptive hemodynamic intervention to improve postoperative outcomes in moderate and high-risk surgical patients. Anesth Analg. 2011;112(6):1392–402.
73. Peng K, Li J, Cheng H, Ji FH. Goal-directed fluid therapy based on stroke volume variations improves fluid management and gastrointestinal perfusion in patients undergoing major orthopedic surgery. Med Princ Pract. 2014;23(5):413–20.
74. Brienza N, Giglio MT, Marucci M, Fiore T. Does perioperative hemodynamic optimization protect renal function in surgical patients? A meta-analytic study. Crit Care Med. 2009;37(6):2079–90.
75. Bacchin MR, Ceria CM, Giannone S, Ghisi D, Stagni G, Greggi T, et al. Goal-directed fluid therapy based on stroke volume variation in patients undergoing major spine surgery in the prone position: a cohort study. Spine. 2016;41(18):E1131–7.
76. Glance LG, Dick AW, Mukamel DB, Fleming FJ, Zollo RA, Wissler R, et al. Association between intraoperative blood transfusion and mortality and morbidity in patients undergoing noncardiac surgery. Anesthesiology. 2011;114(2):283–92.
77. Yuan C, Zhang H, He S. Efficacy and safety of using antifibrinolytic agents in spine surgery: a meta-analysis. PLoS One. 2013;8(11):e82063.
78. Zhang F, Wang K, Li FN, Huang X, Li Q, Chen Z, et al. Effectiveness of tranexamic acid in reducing blood loss in spinal surgery: a meta-analysis. BMC Musculoskelet Disord. 2014;15:448.
79. Cheriyan T, Maier SP 2nd, Bianco K, Slobodyanyuk K, Rattenni RN, Lafage V, et al. Efficacy of tranexamic acid on surgical bleeding in spine surgery: a meta-analysis. Spine J. 2015;15(4):752–61.

Measuring Outcomes in Adult Spinal Deformity

8

Sayf S. A. Faraj, Tsjitske M. Haanstra,
Anna K. Wright, Marinus De Kleuver,
and Miranda L. Van Hooff

The Need for Uniform Outcome Assessment

Several multicenter prospective registries have been created to evaluate quality and value of delivered spine care in population of patients with adult spinal deformity (ASD) [1]. Despite these efforts, global surveillance of patients with ASD and comparative effectiveness of treatment has been hindered by lack of a standardized systematic approach towards outcome measurement and reporting. Although meaningful and valuable for its own local purposes at the originating site, data elements, which are not completely consistent between registries, may not be used for comparison or aggregate analysis as different

S. S. A. Faraj · T. M. Haanstra · M. De Kleuver
Department of Orthopaedic Surgery, Radboud University Nijmegen
Medical Center, Nijmegen, The Netherlands

A. K. Wright
Neuroscience Institute, Virginia Mason Medical Center,
Seattle, WA, USA
e-mail: Anna.Wright@virginiamason.org

M. L. Van Hooff (✉)
Department of Orthopaedic, Radboud University Medical Center,
Nijmegen, The Netherlands

Research, Sint Maartenskliniek, Nijmegen, The Netherlands

© Springer Nature Switzerland AG 2020
R. K. Sethi et al. (eds.), *Value-Based Approaches to Spine Care*,
https://doi.org/10.1007/978-3-030-31946-5_8

outcomes, measurement instruments, and risk stratification variables are used. This inconsistency limits the application of research findings into clinical practice, and prevents clinician investigators from informing policy makers about efficacy of various treatment strategies [2, 3]. One way to address these issues is by developing and implementing an agreed standardized set of treatment outcomes, including a set of (risk) factors that influence these outcomes, also known as a core outcome set (COS). This is a minimum standard set that is recommended for measuring and reporting outcomes in all clinical studies and national outcome registries. Different COSs for several health conditions have already been published and are currently being implemented in routine clinical practice (e.g., for traumatic brain injury and spine trauma) [4, 5].

In a landmark paper, Porter et al. suggested that progress in routine outcome measurement is hampered by the "let a thousand flowers bloom" approach –with each organization reinventing the wheel, tweaking existing measures and risk factors, or inventing one's own [6]. To circumvent this variability, multiple international initiatives have been introduced to bring together researchers who are interested in outcome standardization. These initiatives, including OMERACT (Outcome Measures for Rheumatology Clinical Trials), COMET (Core Outcome Measures in Effectiveness Trials), and ICHOM (International Consortium for Health Outcomes Measurement), provide methodological guidelines for the development of COSs, and add much needed framework for outcome reporting and classification [7, 8].

Low Back Pain Versus ASD

In the case of low back pain (LBP), multiple core outcome sets have been developed using formal consensus methods, such as ICHOM low back pain (LBP) standard outcome set and COS developed by Chiarotto et al. in 2015 [9, 10]. Core areas recommended for inclusion in these outcome sets differ based on the target user, which has implications for the framework used to develop and report each one. For example, the ICHOM LBP set is based on 'what matters to patients', and is aimed at routine outcome measurements to assess the quality of delivered care as part of value-based healthcare initiatives, and for research purposes, whereas the COS was developed for use in clinical trials in low back pain. Currently these COSs have been implemented in multiple (inter-) national spine registries, and have been reported across clinical trials and observational research studies [9–12]. The introduction of these COSs has been essential to the development of a more standardized and systematic approach in measuring and reporting of outcomes in patients with LBP, which is a frequently observed symptom in patients with ASD. However, patients with ASD have significantly other clinical and radiological characteristics than patients with low back pain. For example, neurological and pulmonary function, which is observed to be affected before and after ASD surgery [13, 14], is not included in current standard sets for LBP. Both outcomes could be considered for inclusion in a COS specifically developed for ASD, which makes it necessary to develop a separate COS for ASD that is aligned with the LBP core sets.

Basic Concepts in Outcome Measurement

For the development of a core outcome set, it is important that a universally accepted conceptual framework is used that covers human functioning. The International Classification of Functioning, Disability and Health (ICF) framework, adopted by the World Health Organization, provides the necessary universal language for health outcome measures. More specifically, the ICF framework is intended to describe functional states associated with various health conditions according to a hierarchical classification system [15–17]. Items of (patient-reported and clinician-based) outcome measures can be linked to one or more ICF health outcome domains, depending on the number of meaningful concepts contained in that item (e.g., item 4 of the patient-reported Oswestry Disability Index version 2.1a, "pain does not prevent me from walking any distance", refers to the outcome domains "b280 sensation of pain" and "d450 walking") [18]. Notably, many different health outcomes are currently measured ranging from very generic patient-reported outcome measures (PROMs) to highly disease- and treatment-specific clinician-based measures; each of them have their own purpose for which they were developed.

Prior to the discussion of the process of reaching agreement on a standardized collection of outcomes, it is important to emphasize a basic concept in outcome measurement. A distinction exists between outcome domains, which are defined as the concept or construct to be measured (i.e., pain, walking, self-image) and measurement instruments used to measure these outcome domains (i.e., Visual Analogue Scale, Oswestry Disability Index, and Scoliosis Research Society-22r). A certain outcome domain can be measured using different instruments, which can be categorized into clinician-based or PROMs. For example, the outcome domain "walking" can be measured by using a "6-minute walk" test, which is a clinician-based outcome measurement instrument, or by using a PROM, such as the Oswestry Disability Index. Furthermore, outcome measures can be either 'subjective' – i.e., relying on the interpretation and evaluation by either the patient or by the clinician – or more 'objective', which means independent of the opinion of the observer – e.g., the 6-minute walk test. Note that 'objective' measures do not necessarily mean they are of better methodological quality (e.g., validity or reliability).

Risk Factors and Case-Mix Variables

Benchmarking outcomes is valuable for identifying best practices and in increasing the quality of care [19]. True effects – i.e., improved outcomes that are related to improved quality of care – should be distinguished from improved outcomes that are caused by factors related to the population operated on (e.g., less comorbidity, better pre-operative health), and should not be related to the treatment quality itself. As such, adjustment for patient-related influencing risk factors and case mix variables is required. For example, without this adjustment to the outcomes, patients with more comorbidity would appear to have worse outcomes. When developing a COS it is important not only to reach consensus on the outcomes but also on the pre-treatment risk factors and case-mix variables that could possibly influence the outcome.

What Is a Core Outcome Set?

Benefits

The issue of inconsistent outcome reporting across studies and outcome registries could be addressed by the development and implementation of a COS. This is a consensus-based minimum set of outcome domains, measurement instruments, risk factors and case-mix variables, which should be measured and reported in all clinical studies for a specific disease or disorder [3, 20]. These sets; however, do not imply that outcomes reported should be restricted to those agreed upon in a COS, but rather it is expected that the COS will be collected and reported in future clinical studies and other outcomes or influencing factors can be added that might be of specific interest to researchers, clinicians and institutions. The core outcomes allow for adequate pooling of data and proper comparisons across future clinical studies, systematic reviews, and so-called (national) outcome registries to improve the quality of daily clinical practice.

How to Develop a Core Outcome Set?

Guidelines on COS Development

The COMET initiative, launched in 2010, provides guidelines for the development and application of COSs [21]. The overall aim of COMET is to bring together researchers interested in the development, application and promotion of a COS using rigorous consensus methods. This facilitates the exchange of ideas and information to improve health service users and foster methodological research in the area of standardizing outcomes. Data on current ongoing COS efforts are included in a free, open access repository which is updated periodically [22]. Over the years, there has been a sustained growth in use of the website and database suggesting the gain of interest in the development and implementation of COSs [8].

Scope

Before developing a COS, it is important to agree upon and clearly describe the scope, including details of the health condition, population and type of intervention. It is recommended to check for existing or ongoing development of a COS. Consultation of the database of COMET [www.comet-initiative.org] is recommended to have an overview of the scope and initiatives in the specific area to avoid unnecessary duplication of effort and minimize waste.

Identification of Existing Knowledge

A systematic review of the outcomes (outcome domains and measurement instruments) reported in clinical studies in the area of interest could be used to provide a clear rationale and to explore whether a need exists to develop a COS. In this systematic review current strengths, weaknesses and gaps in outcome assessment in the area of interest could be highlighted and review results could generate a list of potential outcomes to be included in the future COS. To display current outcome domains and measures as reported in eligible studies and to relate to them the concept of human functioning, the ICF framework is frequently used. For example, in a systematic review that provided the preparatory stage of the COS ASD development, outcome domains related to mobility and pain were identified, and were found to be represented by currently used PROMs in the surgical literature of ASD [18]. A gap was identified regarding neurological and pulmonary function, which are known to be affected in the surgical treatment of complex ASD [13, 14]. Both neurological and pulmonary function should be considered for inclusion in the COS, albeit that measuring and reporting of both outcomes have been limited to date.

Stakeholders

Ideally, a COS should include outcomes that are relevant and important to key stakeholders, including patients, health care professionals, researchers, health care policy makers, industry representatives. This means that all relevant stakeholders should be represented when developing a COS using consensus-based methods. The decision on the number of stakeholders from each group is dependent upon the particular scope of the COS as well as practical feasibility considerations. To reach formal consensus, it is recommended to use a method for consensus and to include an uneven number of stakeholders to avoid a tie. If the aim is to develop a COS for global implementation, geographic balance of the consensus panel should be considered as well as the importance of a certain outcome, which might be dependent on cultural and geographical differences.

Consensus Methods

In the development of a COS, the existing knowledge derived from the systematic review in the preparatory stage should be enriched by practice-based knowledge provided by a formal consensus procedure with experts in the specific area of interest. Multiple consensus methods are available, including the (modified) Delphi method [23], Nominal Group Techniques [7], focus groups [24], and individual interviews [25]. The choice of method should be balanced between considerations concerning practicality and ensuring that a diverse range of opinions is heard [22]. A preferred consensus-based method for the development of a COS is the modified Delphi methodology [21]; an iterative process designed to reach formal consensus among a large group of experts using a series of rounds in which participants vote on or rate statements. In the case of a COS: e.g., in- or exclusion of certain outcomes. A predefined threshold for consensus is determined – e.g., 75% equal votes. The Delphi process is anonymous to make sure all participants have an equal say. After each round, stakeholders receive anonymous feedback report of the group's ratings to reflect on these outcomes and rate outcomes again where no consensus was reached. Often in the final round, stakeholders are invited to meet face-to-face to review the Delphi findings and discuss the COS in a formal setting led by an independent moderator to reach a final consensus. In general, formal consensus is reached on outcome domains (i.e., 'what' should be measured), after which consensus is reached on the measurement instruments ('how' to measure the outcome domains), as well as time-points for assessment.

Challenges in the Development of a COS

The development of a COS is an important step towards a standardized and systematic outcome measurement reporting for a specific health condition. It will not achieve its goal if reports of the COS are not complete and transparent. The Core Outcome Set–STAndards for Reporting (COS-STAR) statement is a published checklist of 18 items considered essential for transparent and complete reporting in all COS studies [26]. This checklist supports the completeness in the report of a COS, which future users can use to judge whether the recommended standard set is relevant for their population of interest. Consideration should be given in advance to other challenges when developing a COS. Pre-selection of stakeholders (by personal invitation) to participate in the development of a COS may increase the risk of selection bias, and may result in a COS that is not applicable to all cultures. As such, participation of a patient panel and validation in international patient-focus groups needs to be considered. Moreover, inconclusive or undefined concepts can be encountered during identification of potential core outcome domains for which no measurement instruments exist and are yet to be developed. After completion of a COS sufficient attention should be given to dissemination and implementation.

Core Outcome Set for ASD

Routine outcome measurement is challenging but when implemented successfully it has many benefits. For example, research has shown that asking providers to measure and report outcomes alone already improves performance [27]. Understanding and comparing outcomes facilitates continuous learning and improvement of own strategies through learning from best practices. Continuous improvement and informed decision-making could be important driving forces in improving the quality of healthcare delivery by for example value-based healthcare. This may specifically be beneficial for complex clinical entities such as ASD where randomized controlled trials (RCTs) are often not practical, ethically challenging, and for which a tremendous variability in management strategies exists. Given the expanding interest in patient-centered care and increasing treatment costs, a systematic and standardized approach towards routine outcome assessment by means of a COS for ASD is of utmost importance in the era towards value-based healthcare. This will subsequently allow for intentional data pooling and benchmarking of outcomes, and in turn highlight the value of provided (surgical) treatment.

The development of a COS for ASD has been initiated by the Scoliosis Research Society (SRS) and is currently under development. The scope is ASD patients over 25 years of age undergoing surgical or non-surgical treatment. A modified Delphi study is currently being performed. The working group includes a total of 25 stakeholders from across the world that had to meet strict membership requirements of the SRS [28], which includes the ability to demonstrate their interest in spine deformity (e.g., attend annual meetings, and submit and review abstracts), and at least 5 years of experience in spine deformity surgery or research. A project team not participating in the Delphi rounds is guiding and coordinating the efforts of the larger working group of panelists.

In preparation for the Delphi study, the project team performed a structured systematic literature review to identify currently used outcomes and outcome measurement instruments in the surgical literature of ASD [18]. Identified outcomes were classified within the World Health Organization's International Classification of Functioning, Disability and Health (WHO-ICF). The literature review included 144 papers on ASD surgery and yielded a list of 29 ICF outcomes, which was used as the foundation for consensus rounds. A list with potential risk factors and case-mix variables that could influence the treatment outcome and should be included in the COS was derived from multiple published sources,

Table 8.1 (continued)

	Patient-reported	Clinician-reported
Pre-operative clinical status		BMI 21; non-smoker; no previous spine surgery; co-morbidities: ASA II
Surgical procedure		Primary surgery; 1-stage procedure; Posterolateral instrumented fusion – 8 levels + pelvic fixation; OR time 253 minutes; LoS: 5 days

ODI v2.1a Oswestry Disability Index version 2.1a (0–100; functional status), *SRS22r* Scoliosis Research Society 22 revised version (1–5; condition-specific health-related quality of life), *EQ5D-3 L* EuroQol 5 Dimensions with 3 answer categories (−0.125–1.000; health related quality of life), *VAS* Visual Analogue Scale (0–100), *NPRS* Numeric Pain Rating Scale (0–10; current pain intensity), *OR* Operating Room – knife time, *LoS* Length of hospital stay

Table 8.2 Case example: Outcomes *1 year after surgery*

	Patient-reported		Clinician-reported
Tier 1 Health status achieved or retained Survival			
Degree of health or recovery	ODI v2.1a: 36 SRS22r:		
	Function	4.0	
	Pain	4.2	
	Self-image	4.2	
	Mental health	4.4	
	Satisfaction	4.6	
	Total	4.3	
	EQ5D-3 L:		
	Utility	0.775	
	VAS	65/100	
	NPRS:		
	Back	3/10	
	Leg	2/10	

(continued)

Table 8.2 (continued)

	Patient-reported	Clinician-reported
Tier 2 Process of recovery		
Time to recovery & time to return to normal activities	Return to work: 22 weeks (part-time)	
Disutility of care or treatment process		No complications during hospital stay
Tier 3 Sustainability of health		
Sustainability of health or recovery and nature of recurrences		No revision surgery needed
Long-term consequences of treatment		Development of Proximal Junctional Kyphosis (PJK)

ODI v2.1a Oswestry Disability Index version 2.1a (0–100; functional status), *SRS22r* Scoliosis Research Society 22 revised version (1–5; condition-specific health-related quality of life), *EQ5D-3 L* EuroQol 5 Dimensions with 3 answer categories (−0.125–1.000; health related quality of life), *VAS* Visual Analogue Scale (0–100), *NPRS* Numeric Pain Rating Scale (0–10; current pain intensity)

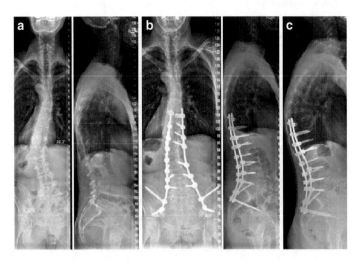

Fig. 8.1 Case example: (**a**) Pre-operative, (**b**) Post-operative, and (**c**) One-year follow-up full spine radiographs. Development of Proximal Junctional Kyphosis (PJK) shown at one-year follow-up assessment

When implemented, this standard set allows for monitoring and meaningful comparisons of risk-adjusted surgical outcomes in ASD across (inter-) national institutions, studies, and spine registries to improve the quality of care delivered in daily clinical practice. Ultimately, it could enhance outcome measurement to determine the value of treatment provided for patients with ASD.

References

1. van Hooff ML, Jacobs WCH, Willems PC, et al. Evidence and practice in spine registries. Acta Orthop. 2015;86:534–44. https://doi.org/10.3109/1 7453674.2015.1043174.
2. Williamson P, Altman D, Blazeby J, et al. Driving up the quality and relevance of research through the use of agreed core outcomes. J Health Serv Res Policy. 2012;17:1–2.
3. Clarke M. Standardising outcomes for clinical trials and systematic reviews. Trials. 2007;8:39. https://doi.org/10.1186/1745-6215-8-39.
4. Oner FC, Jacobs WCH, Lehr AM, et al. Toward the development of a universal outcome instrument for spine trauma: a systematic review and content comparison of outcome measures used in spine trauma research using the ICF as reference. Spine (Phila Pa 1976). 2016;41:358–67. https://doi.org/10.1097/BRS.0000000000001207.
5. Laxe S, Tschiesner U, Zasler N, et al. What domains of the International Classification of Functioning, Disability and Health are covered by the most commonly used measurement instruments in traumatic brain injury research? Clin Neurol Neurosurg. 2012;114:645–50. https://doi.org/10.1016/j.clineuro.2011.12.038.
6. Porter ME, Larsson S, Lee TH. Standardizing patient outcomes measurement. N Engl J Med. 2016;374:504–6. https://doi.org/10.1056/NEJMp1511701.
7. Tugwell P, Boers M, Brooks P, et al. OMERACT: an international initiative to improve outcome measurement in rheumatology. Trials. 2007;8:38. https://doi.org/10.1186/1745-6215-8-38.
8. Gargon E, Williamson PR, Altman DG, et al. The COMET Initiative database: progress and activities update (2015). Trials. 2017;18:54. https://doi.org/10.1186/s13063-017-1788-8.
9. Chiarotto A, Deyo RA, Terwee CB, et al. Core outcome domains for clinical trials in non-specific low back pain. Eur Spine J. 2015;24:1127–42. https://doi.org/10.1007/s00586-015-3892-3.
10. Clement RC, Welander A, Stowell C, et al. A proposed set of metrics for standardized outcome reporting in the management of low back pain. Acta Orthop. 2015;86:1–11. https://doi.org/10.3109/17453674.2015.103 6696.

11. Deyo RA, Battie M, Beurskens AJ, et al. Outcome measures for low back pain research. A proposal for standardized use. Spine (Phila Pa 1976). 1998;23:2003–13.
12. Deyo RA, Dworkin SF, Amtmann D, et al. Report of the NIH Task Force on research standards for chronic low back pain. Phys Ther. 2015;95:e1–e18. https://doi.org/10.2522/ptj.2015.95.2.e1.
13. Lenke LG, Fehlings MG, Shaffrey CI, et al. Neurologic outcomes of complex adult spinal deformity surgery: results of the prospective, multicenter Scoli-RISK-1 study. Spine (Phila Pa 1976). 2016;41:204–12. https://doi.org/10.1097/BRS.0000000000001338.
14. Lehman RA, Kang DG, Lenke LG, et al. Pulmonary function following adult spinal deformity surgery: minimum two-year follow-up. J Bone Joint Surg Am. 2015;97:32–9. https://doi.org/10.2106/JBJS.N.00408.
15. WHO. International classification of functioning, disability and health. Geneva: World Health Organization; 2001.
16. Cieza A, Stucki G, Weigl M, et al. ICF Core Sets for low back pain. J Rehabil Med. 2004;36:69–74. https://doi.org/10.1080/16501960410016037.
17. Stucki G, Cieza A, Melvin J. The International Classification of Functioning, Disability and Health (ICF): a unifying model for the conceptual description of the rehabilitation strategy. J Rehabil Med. 2007;39:279–85. https://doi.org/10.2340/16501977-0041.
18. Faraj SSA, van Hooff ML, Holewijn RM, et al. Measuring outcomes in adult spinal deformity surgery: a systematic review to identify current strengths, weaknesses and gaps in patient-reported outcome measures. Eur Spine J. 2017;26:2084–93. https://doi.org/10.1007/s00586-017-5125-4.
19. Spence RT, Mueller JL, Chang DC. A novel approach to global benchmarking of risk-adjusted surgical outcomes: beyond perioperative mortality rate. JAMA Surg. 2016;151:501–2. https://doi.org/10.1001/jamasurg.2016.0091.
20. Boonen A, Braun J, van der Horst Bruinsma IE, et al. ASAS/WHO ICF Core Sets for ankylosing spondylitis (AS): how to classify the impact of AS on functioning and health. Ann Rheum Dis. 2010;69:102–7. https://doi.org/10.1136/ard.2008.104117.
21. Prinsen CAC, Vohra S, Rose MR, et al. Core Outcome Measures in Effectiveness Trials (COMET) initiative: protocol for an international Delphi study to achieve consensus on how to select outcome measurement instruments for outcomes included in a "core outcome set". Trials. 2014;15:247. https://doi.org/10.1186/1745-6215-15-247.
22. Williamson PR, Altman DG, Blazeby JM, et al. Developing core outcome sets for clinical trials: issues to consider. Trials. 2012;13:132. https://doi.org/10.1186/1745-6215-13-132.
23. Schmitt J, Langan S, Stamm T, Williams HC. Core outcome domains for controlled trials and clinical recordkeeping in eczema: international multiperspective Delphi consensus process. J Invest Dermatol. 2011;131:623–30. https://doi.org/10.1038/jid.2010.303.

24. Sanderson T, Morris M, Calnan M, et al. What outcomes from pharmacologic treatments are important to people with rheumatoid arthritis? Creating the basis of a patient core set. Arthritis Care Res (Hoboken). 2010;62:640–6. https://doi.org/10.1002/acr.20034.

25. Kirwan J, Heiberg T, Hewlett S, et al. Outcomes from the Patient Perspective Workshop at OMERACT 6. J Rheumatol. 2003;30:868–72.

26. Kirkham JJ, Gorst S, Altman DG, et al. Core outcome set–STAndards for reporting: the COS-STAR statement. PLoS Med. 2016;13:e1002148. https://doi.org/10.1371/journal.pmed.1002148.

27. Porter M. What is value in health care? N Engl J Med. 2010;2477–81. https://doi.org/10.1056/NEJMp1415160.

28. Scoliosis Research Society Membership. Accessed 28-02-2018. http://www.srs.org/professionals/membership.

29. Lapp MA, Bridwell KH, Lenke LG, et al. Long-term complications in adult spinal deformity patients having combined surgery: a comparison of primary of revision patients. Spine (Phila Pa 1976). 2001;26:973–83.

30. Pull ter Gunne AF, van Laarhoven CJHM, Cohen DB, et al. Incidence of surgical site infection following adult spinal deformity surgery: an analysis of patient risk. Eur Spine J. 2010;19:982–8. https://doi.org/10.1007/s00586-009-1269-1.

31. Soroceanu A, Diebo BG, Burton D, et al. Radiographical and implant-related complications in adult spinal deformity surgery. Spine (Phila Pa 1976).2015;40:1414–21.https://doi.org/10.1097/BRS.0000000000001020.

32. Carreon LY, Glassman SD, Shaffrey CI, et al. Predictors of health-related quality-of-life after complex adult spinal deformity surgery: a Scoli-RISK-1 secondary analysis. Spine Deform. 2017;5:139–44. https://doi.org/10.1016/j.jspd.2016.11.001.

33. Pellisé F, Vila-Casademunt A, Núñez-Pereira S, et al. The Adult Deformity Surgery Complexity Index (ADSCI): a valid tool to quantify the complexity of posterior adult spinal deformity surgery and predict postoperative complications. Spine J. 2018;18:216–25. https://doi.org/10.1016/j.spinee.2017.06.042.

34. Leven DM, Lee NJ, Kothari P, et al. Frailty index is a significant predictor of complications and mortality after surgery for adult spinal deformity. Spine (Phila Pa 1976). 2016;41:E1394–401. https://doi.org/10.1097/BRS.0000000000001886.

35. Scheer JK, Smith JS, Schwab F, et al. Development of a preoperative predictive model for major complications following adult spinal deformity surgery. J Neurosurg Spine. 2017;26:736–43. https://doi.org/10.3171/2016.10.SPINE16197.

36. Pull ter Gunne AF, Hosman AJF, Cohen DB, et al. A methodological systematic review on surgical site infections following spinal surgery. Spine (Phila Pa1976).2012;37:2017–33.https://doi.org/10.1097/BRS.0b013e31825bfca8.

37. Baron EM, Albert TJ. Medical complications of surgical treatment of adult spinal deformity and how to avoid them. Spine (Phila Pa 1976). 2006;31:S106–18. https://doi.org/10.1097/01.brs.0000232713.69342.df.
38. Di Capua J, Somani S, Kim JS, et al. Hospital-acquired conditions in adult spinal deformity surgery: predictors for hospital-acquired conditions and other 30-day postoperative outcomes. Spine (Phila Pa 1976). 2017;42:595–602. https://doi.org/10.1097/BRS.0000000000001840.
39. Manoharan SR, Baker DK, Pasara SM, et al. Thirty-day readmissions following adult spinal deformity surgery: an analysis of the National Surgical Quality Improvement Program (NSQIP) database. Spine J. 2016;16:862–6. https://doi.org/10.1016/j.spinee.2016.03.014.

Spine Safety: Optimum Integration of Technology

9

Richard Menger, Han Jo Kim, and Michael G. Vitale

Technological advances in the field of spine surgery have facilitated the delivery of effective and safe treatments for a wide range of spinal diseases. These technologies enable spine surgeons to safely and efficiently treat even the most complex spinal disorders. Robotic surgical assistance, spinal instrumentation advances, computer-assisted operative navigation, intra-operative computed tomography, real-time neuromonitoring, and minimally invasive techniques are some of the technologies that will be evaluated in this chapter.

R. Menger
Department of Neurosurgery, New York-Presbyterian Hospital-Columbia and Cornell, New York, NY, USA

H. J. Kim
Department of Orthopaedic, Hospital for Special Surgery, New York, NY, USA

M. G. Vitale (✉)
Pediatric Spine and Scoliosis Service, Division of Pediatric Orthopaedic, Quality & Strategy, Orthopaedic Surgery, Columbia University Medical Center/Morgan Stanley Children's Hospital, New York, NY, USA
e-mail: mgv1@cumc.columbia.edu

© Springer Nature Switzerland AG 2020
R. K. Sethi et al. (eds.), *Value-Based Approaches to Spine Care*,
https://doi.org/10.1007/978-3-030-31946-5_9

Technologies enhance the efficacy of spine surgery and have even made certain surgeries possible where historically they simply could not be done. Yet, the vital distinction remains that the safety of the procedure is primarily the surgeon's responsibility. The surgeon must be a proper integrator and adaptor of technological developments. Surgeons must use the technologies only as a tool to assist in the procedure and not as a substitute for surgical experience, meticulous attention to detail, or clinical objectiveness that are critical for achieving favorable outcomes. This chapter provides an in-depth analysis of these technologies, and assesses their impact on improving safety and in spinal surgery.

Technology Adoption Life Cycle

As a way into this topic, it is important that surgeons understand the overarching framework regarding the adoption of technological advancements. Historically in 1962, Rogers et al. introduced the *Diffusion of Innovations Theory* as it applied to farming technology. Of the population, 2.5% will be innovators, 13.5% early adopters, 34% early majority, 34% later majority, and 16% laggards in standard bell curve type format. This concept piece has diffused into cancer prevention, communication, and even drunk driving prevention. The idea is that innovators are generally extremely educated thought leaders who are prosperous in their community and very risk-oriented. Often, no marketing or positioning is needed to "convince" this population to adopt a technology. Early adopters tend to be younger emerging community thought leaders. They understand that to remain relevant as an opinion leader, they must adopt a cycle of change. The early majority are generally the cohort conservatively open to new ideas and are in a position to influence the decision-making of others but on a lesser scale. The late majority tend to be less socially active and skeptical of change while laggards are very conservative and respond very rigidly to only statistics, logic, and evidence from earlier adoption groups [1].

Self-awareness of the surgeon into which category they fall into is vitally important for the proper integration of technology that could specifically improve patient outcomes. Early adopters and innovators will have a different complication profile with emerging technology than laggards or the late majority. The innovators will undoubtedly have more early-onset technological problems or glitches as new technology is adapted. This can be seen in some of the frustrations around first generation technology of any kind. Frustrations regarding robotic surgery technology immediately come to mind. Meanwhile, laggards are positioned to possibly see old techniques and old tools as providing a greater complication profile than new technology. An example of this would be a neurosurgeon who refuses to use cranial CT navigation for the placement of a ventriculo-peritoneal shunt in the setting of slit ventricles [2].

Advances in Spinal Instrumentation

Prior to the widespread use of innovative technologies in the field of spine surgery, surgeons were limited in their ability to correct spinal pathology. The procedures of surgical reconstruction of the spinal column included the use of sub-laminar wires, challenging pelvic fixation devices, and posterior element hooks. These early techniques did show success but at an inconsistent level with different biomechanical disadvantages [3–6]. These historical corrective approaches gave the surgeon a very limited control of the spine. During complex spinal deformity surgery for example, it is extremely advantageous for surgeons to have precise control over the position of individual spinal segments in all three columns. Currently, pedicle screws are the technological advancement that allows for this exact type of control and precision. Dr. Harrington was the first surgeon to describe the process of placing screws down the long axis of the pedicle in his 1965 report that utilized this technology in the treatment of how high-grade spondylolisthesis in children [7]. Roy-Camile also published a paper in 1970 describing this technique and giving a formal presentation at the 1979 American Academy of Orthopedic Surgeons Annual Meeting [8]. Professor Suk introduced thoracic pedicle screws as a segmental technique for spinal deformity proving them to be both safe and effective. Since then, pedicle screws have emerged as the mainstay of posterior spinal fixation allowing for precise control and greater manipulation of the spinal column than traditional laminar hooks and wires.

Because of pedicle screw instrumentation, and the control over the three columns of the spine that it can provide, there has been a general shift to posterior-only approaches in complex spine surgery. Posterior column osteotomies, vertebral column resections, and pedicle-subtraction osteotomies, can be done with increased safety because pedicle screws have afforded surgeons greater control and manipulation of the spine. Thanks to these procedures, surgeons are able to rectify serious spinal deformities that would have otherwise been untreatable a few decades ago [9–11]. This is vividly illustrated through national case selection trends. The incidence of aggressive deformity correction surgery is increasing rapidly. From 2008 to 2011, there was a 246% increase in the use of pedicle subtraction osteotomy in national Medicare data [12]. Even as the trend to more harmonious correction is currently developing, posterior-centric construction is the mainstay of corrective techinques [13]. This, at least in part, can be due to improved instrumentation capability.

Neuromonitoring

The ability to monitor the status of the spinal cord and specifically the neural elements in real time during spine surgery has greatly enhanced the patient's safety. Major developments have occurred in the past two decades [14]. Neuromonitoring is not only limited to complex spine operations and can be employed even in minor spine surgeries to avoid inadvertent neurologic injury.

The three major pillars of intra-operative neuromonitoring are somatosensory-evoked potentials (SSEPs), trans-cranial motor-evoked potentials (MEPs), and electromyography (EMG). The SSEPs are highly specific in detecting spinal cord injury during surgery, and they do this by stimulating the peripheral nerves and recording the corresponding electrical potential with trans-cranial sensors. Surgeons are then able to assess the integrity and functions of the dorsal sensory column based on these recordings [14]. MEPs, compared to SSEPs, are less specific, but can detect neurologic injury better since they directly monitor the spinal cord's motor pathway by recording the response of specific peripheral muscles when the cranial motor cortex is stimulated. Electrodes placed into the scalp stimulate the motor cortex to directly evaluate the spinal cord pyramidal tracts [14]. The data obtained from SSEPs and MEPs affords the surgeon with real time information on the status of the spinal cord and its sensory and motor functions.

The surgeon is typically notified when the SSEPs have a unilateral (or bilateral) reduction in amplitude of 50–60% or a 10% increase in latency [14]. MEP "hits" focus on either a threshold technique, amplitude technique, or all or none technique [14].

Electromyography provides more direct information regarding the spontaneous electrical activity of muscles and therefore nerve root level innervation. They can be monitored in either a spontaneous or triggered fashion. Spontaneous EMG markings obtain baseline EMGs at the start of the case to obtain a baseline activity level of a "quiet" or unstimulated muscles without any nerve root irritation. Significant burst pattern changes leading to non-repetitive asynchronous potentials or train activity may indicate nerve root irritation or damage during the procedure [14].

Triggered EMGs (tEMGs) use electrical stimulation in a targeted fashion to evaluate pedicle screw breaches. A lower stimulation suggests a cortical breach in the bone of the pedicle that allows the triggered stimulation to record activity the paraspinal musculature. A threshold of 10 V has a sensitivity of 94% and 90% of determining pedicle screw malposition resulting in a breach of the cortical wall [14].

Numerous spine specific literature illustrate that when interpreted correctly, intra-operative neuromonitoring is both sensitive and specific in detecting neurologic compromise. The sensitivity is reported at 90–95% and specificity at 96–99% [15–18]. Fehling et al., for instance, reviewed literature with high quality studies that reinforced the notion that trans-cranial motor neuromonitoring is both sensitive and specific for detecting neurologic injury in real time [19]. It tends to be the most sensitive for modality for spinal cord injury [14]. This allows for information that can result in a different surgical intervention that can make a difference in clinical outcome. Monitoring the status of the spinal cord during surgery in real time does enhance the safety of the procedure and allows for the surgeon to reverse deformity correction, explore nerve roots of otherwise occult compression, and continue searching for potential causes for a neurologic deficit that may have otherwise been overlooked until it is too late to be rectified.

Consequently, best practice guidelines have been developed by Vitale et al. to standardize and maximize response to changes in neuromonitoring that occur intraoperatively. This can be found in Fig. 9.1. The checklist involves a multidisciplinary approach with several team members in a stepwise fashion. However, the driving force behind this safety mechanism is the technology of intraoperative neuromonitoring.

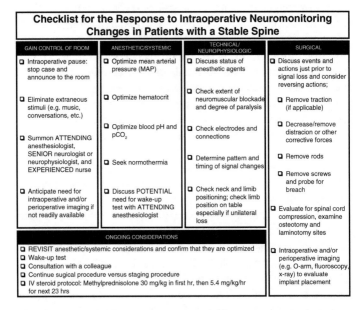

Fig. 9.1 Checklist for response to neuromonitoring changes. (From Vitale et al. [51], with permission)

It is important that surgeons understand that this technology is not a substitute for clinical judgment. The overwhelming majority of literature illustrates that neuromonitoring can provide the surgical team with both sensitive and specific info regarding the patient's neurologic status. However, several initial publications have described instances where the intra-operative neuromonitoring data came back as "normal' whereas the patient suffered significant neurologic deficits. This has been observed mostly in cases where the surgical team relied only on SSEPs data [20–22]. There are also relatively infrequent instances of false positives whereby data from intra-neuromonitoring techniques indicate a negative neurologic status yet the patient awakens with normal sensory and motor functions – which are reported at around 5–8% [23]. The key is to have a standardized integrated team using multiple platforms including SSEP, MEP, and EMG. This breaks into the notion of, in order to be safe, the surgeon must understand, integrate, and use the proper leading technology.

Again, a constant theme, this information is an adjunct to the surgeon's clinical decision. Technology is not a substitute. It merely provides more information to the surgeon to improve the safety of surgery. The surgeon must integrate this information with expertise, clinical-decision making, and a standardized-response format. Ignoring a change in neuromonitoring can be disastrous, but this has very different implications for an elective anterior cervical discectomy with fusion as compared to the non-ambulatory neuromuscular scoliosis with multiple medical co-morbidities.

Minimally Invasive Surgical (MIS) Techniques

Minimally invasive surgical (MIS) approaches are mainly utilized to ensure patients incur minimal damage to soft tissues during surgery. The MIS technique has several specific advantages including decreased muscle and tendon stripping, muscle function preservation and integrity, less blood loss, and smaller incisions. MIS techniques have also been reported to improve patient safety since it potentially lowers the infection rates, and the time to recovery aftersurgery [24, 25].

MIS and Safety in Spine

Adongwa et al. demonstrated that patients who underwent MIS trans-foraminal lumbar interbody fusion (TLIF), as opposed to open TLIF, had shorter hospital stay (3 vs. 5.5 days), decreased duration of narcotics post-op (2 vs. 4 weeks), and resumed work faster (8.5 vs. 17 weeks). Both groups showed similar improvements in pain and back related disability at 2 years [26]. This has significant patient and societal cost-related impact. Results of a meta-analysis comparing open TLIF to MIS TLIF showed that the latter has less blood loss, and since the intra- and post-operative transfusion rates were not availed, it could not be determined whether the differences were clinically significant. What was confirmed, however, was that both approaches (open TLIF and MIS TLIF) had similar re-operation rates, operative times, and complication rates [27]. Moreover, other studies have confirmed similar operative time (182 minutes Open TLIF, 166 minutes MIS, $p > 0.05$), less blood loss (447 ml vs. 50 ml), longer fluoroscopic time (17.6 s open, 49 s MIS), less morphine requirements (33.5 mg open vs. 3.4 mg MIS), less post-operative drainage (open 528 ml, MIS 0 ml), and shorter hospital stay (6.8 days open, 3.2 days MIS) with MIS surgery. Additionally, similar improvements for visual analogue pain scale improvement, overall health improvement on the Short-Form 36 (SF-36) questionnaires, Oswestry Disability Index (ODI), and similar fusion rates between both groups at 2 years (98 vs. 97%) for both groups [28, 29].

Adverse events in open- and MIS lumbar fusion have been analyzed using large meta-analysis and systematic reviews. In a study comparing 806 open patients and 856 MIS patients, the results showed MIS fusion was associated with lower blood loss (260 ml less), 3.5 days faster time to 'normal' ambulation, and shorter hospitalization (2.9 days) [30]. In the meta-analysis, there was no difference in intra-operative complications, operative time, or adverse events. Additionally, between MIS and open lumbar fusion, there was no significant difference noted in non-union or revision surgery rates. MIS cases were significantly less likely to experience medical adverse events (risk ratio [MIS vs. open] = 0.39, 95% confidence interval 0.23–0.69, $p = 0.001$).

However, it is important to note some nuances of the data. All studies included in the meta-analysis were considered to be low or very low quality with inherent bias. This remains an interest and important evolving field within spine surgery.

While the science of minimally invasive spine surgery is progressing and evolving to improve outcomes and patient safety, it comes with a steep learning curve. Investigation has clearly indicated that surgeons find it quite challenging to master MIS techniques because they require in-depth understanding of the anatomy of the spine and exemplary three-dimensional spatial-visual skills [31]. The learning curve can be even be steep with experienced surgeons. Nevertheless, it is proven in a peer-reviewed format that MIS techniques reduces hospital stays, lower infection rate, has less blood loss, and provides faster recovery time.

It is important to recognize the synergy of technological advancement that has allowed MIS techniques to flourish. An electronically moveable radiolucent operating table, the ability to use high-quality fluoroscopy intraoperatively, and the ability to now integrate intra-operative navigation of CT scans are just a sample. However, it remains important that surgeons again remain in realistic ownership of the operative theatre and operative outcome. That is, true MIS surgery requires a learning curve and a safety paradigm that is somewhat different for each surgeon. There is a tremendous difference in undertaking technology guided advancement for better patient outcomes and a competition-based marketing approach relying technological adjuncts.

Intra-Operative CT and Three-Dimensional Navigation

As outlined earlier in the chapter, pedicle screws are an indispensable asset to a spine surgeon, but only if they are safely inserted. And, pedicle screw insertion can be challenging, despite widespread adoption, breaches can still occur. The key to the safe placement of the pedicle screw is contingent on the surgeon's comprehension of the dorsal spine bony anatomy and the relative orientation of the pedicle in relation to the posterior column [32]

Not only should surgeons be knowledgeable on the landmarks that define the dorsal anatomy, they also need to be familiar with the three-dimensional orientation of pedicles at each level in the spine. Pedicle screws should be accurately placed within the bony channel of the pedicle to ensure maximum pullout strength of the screw, avoid neurologic injury, leakage of the cerebrospinal fluid, and spinal cord or nerve root irritation.

Studies have reported significant variations in accuracy levels of plain radiographs and intra-operative fluoroscopy in determining pedicle screw placement. A study by Parker et al. reported a pedicle breach rate of 1.7% of pedicle screws placed using true free-hand technique and the radiographs obtained after the screw is in place [33]. Based on reports from several meta-analyses, spine experts generally agree that pedicle screw malposition rate is around 10–15% [34]. Several factors, such as differences in surgical experience and technique, limitations of fluoroscopy, and limitations of 2-dimensional assessment to accurately assess screw placement into a pedicle, can be partially used to elucidate the difference in variation rates [35].

As such, intraoperative CT and 3D navigation of have developed to support improved accuracy of pedicle screw placement. These are two separate adjuncts that can be linked into application. Compared to plain radiography, computerized-tomography (CT) is much more sensitive in assessing the accuracy of pedicle screw placement [36]. Thus, the introduction of intra-operative CT technology in posterior spinal fixation procedures can greatly enhance the process in such a way that surgeons can accurately determine pedicle screw placement during the immediate intraoperative course. Surgeons are able to reposition misaligned screws without having to perform another surgery on the patient. As the intra-operative CT scans continue to evolve, they may be coupled with computer navigation technology, which gives the surgery team a live, real-life view of the pedicle and cannulation tools in the axial, sagittal, and coronal plane. This technology creates a variety of technological workflows for the spine surgeon. It allows the CT imaging platform to function as an adjunct of confirmation after free-hand or fluoroscopic guided placement of pedicle screws or as direct CT guidance.

Empirical data confirms that computer-assisted navigation technology enhances safety in spinal instrumentation by increasing accuracy. A systematic and meta-analysis of spine literature indicates that, compared to the other methods of assessing the accuracy of pedicle screw placement, instances of pedicle violation was much lower when the surgical team used CT-based navigation systems to determine if the screws were accurately placed (Odds ratio 0.32–0.60, $p < 0.01$) [37]. At the margins, there are reports of accurate pedicle cannulation in 68% of "convectional" cases as compared to 95% accuracy when navigation technology was utilized in the procedure [36].

It is important to also recognize the challenge in comparing different modalities for the accurate placement of pedicle screws. Variations in the reported accuracy of the free-hand technique may be the likely difference between surgeons in terms of surgical capabilities and operative experience. A novice surgeon may report a larger discrepancy in accuracy between free-hand and navigated techniques of placing pedicle screws as compared to a surgeon with many years of experience whose variation between the two techniques might not show a large difference. Therefore, it can be argued that CT-navigation closes the gap separating experienced surgeons from the novices-novice surgeons [38]. Each surgeon must integrate technology at the appropriate level for their practice. As per theme, technology should be integrated into technical mastery but substituted for it.

This creates an open challenge to academic surgeons and surgeons-in-training. As navigational systems become more ubiquitous, it remains vitally important that senior mentors and trainees take an active role to remain fluent in free-hand and fluoroscopic techniques. Technology works with the surgeon and not for the surgeon. It is obvious that, as is the case with every technological surgical tool, CT-navigation works best in situations with the highest level of competency, sound clinical judgment and careful attention to details on the part of the surgical team. The surgeon cannot maximize patient's safety when these attributes are missing in the operating room. The surgeon must be prepared when (not if) the technology stops working.

In summation, intraoperative CT imaging and navigation are valuable technological adjuncts. Both have been illustrated to be both effective and safe. Each individual surgeon must best develop a technological integration platform that fits their needs and the realities of their hospital and local community practice.

Robotic Spine Surgery

Surgeons in all field, are now pivoting to robotic surgery in an effort to increase efficiency and safety. In spine surgery, for instance, techniques such as the robotic-assisted pedicle cannulation was developed to assist in quick and accurate placement of pedicle screws using both open and MIS techniques. Using a pre-operative CT scan, this technology is able to first create a digital "map" of the patient's spinal anatomy; then as the surgical team begins the procedure, they obtain fluoroscopic radiographs, which are juxtaposed by the robotic software on the CT scan to determine where the elements of the spinal cord are in space. A reference point is then secured on the patient and the surgeon is then guided by a robotic arm to the correct starting point and the trajectory of the desired pedicle. The surgeon uses the Seldinger technique to drill into the pedicle and place a guide wire, tap the screws to the desired caliber, and finally insert the pedicle screw. In theory, this procedure should be quite effective at reducing large discrepancies in accurate placement of pedicle screws among surgeons while enhancing patient's safety. When compared to CT navigation the robotic technology is able to use a segmental navigation points that aren't interrupted by wholesale changes to spinal anatomy or navigation.

Several studies have examined the accuracy of robot-assisted pedicle screw cannulation. For example, a retrospective study by Kantelhardt et al. in 2011 established that 94.5% of pedicle screws that were placed with the guidance of robotic arms were accurately placed as compared with the success rate of 91.4% in the freehand group, a statistical significant difference. The same study also found no significant difference in accuracy when it compared the application of the robotic arm in both percutaneous and open (midline incision) screw placement [39]. Schatlo et al., using the Gertzbein-robbins classification, reported 83.6% "perfect" placement in robotic insertion compared to 79% with freehand technique [39, 40]. New studies continue to demonstrate high accuracy rate in robotic cohorts, ranging from 85% to nearly 100%, of robotic-assisted pedicle and S2-Alar-illiac cannulation [41–43]. Meanwhile, Gao and Yu do not concur with these reports via their meta-analyses and systematic reviews concede that the available evidence is hardly enough to determine the superiority of robotic pedicle cannulation over other placement techniques such as CT-Navigation and the freehand [44, 45]. Indeed, the debate is in its primary stages regarding the accuracy of robotic assisted cannulation. Larger and systematic studies need to be undertaken to compare this technology with more conventional approaches to pedicle placement.

An interesting caveat to this technology is that it allows the surgical team to precisely plan the pedicle screw start point and essentially avoid violating the superior facet joint in fusion constructs, which in turn may decrease iatrogenic instability of the adjacent level. Kim et al. proved that indeed this was the case in their randomized trial of free-hand versus robot-assisted pedicle screw fixation. From their study, they observed that although there was hardly any perceivable difference in accuracy of pedicle cannulation, but the robotic sample enjoyed a 0% superior facet violations compared to the 15% reported in the open freehand group [46]. These findings by Kim et al. have been corroborated by Gao et al. in their meta-analysis of robotic freehand screw placement [44]. It is imperative to understand that the benefits associated with bypassing the cephalad facet joint with pedicle screw placement and are only theoretical. Park et al. established that there were no differences in clinical outcomes or adjustment segment degeneration after studying two-year results of MIS-Robotic fusion patients compared to freehand fusion techniques, despite fewer facet violations in the robotic-assisted group [47]. Park et al. admit that their sample size for the study was limited and consequently they cannot authoritatively determine whether or not the cranial facet avoidance is clinically relevant.

Another advantageous application of robotic-assisted spine instrumentation is that it reduces the amount of radiation being exposed by the surgical team and the patient in the operating room, thereby enhancing safety. This can be non-trivial, especially in MIS cases. Using the same meta-analysis that assessed both robotic and freehand techniques Gao and Yu illustrated the radiation difference between the two techniques. These studies associated robot-assisted pedicle cannulation with reduced radiation time (mean difference = 12.38). The radiation dosage exposed to the surgeon was also significantly lower (64% less). Obviously, the amount of fluoroscopy is variable by surgeon and surgeon technique.

Spine literature notes that robotic instrumentation technology can be of tremendous benefit in the situations of distorted spinal anatomy. Placement of instrumentation through either severe deformity or previous fusion mass can be extremely challenging. Robotic surgery can serve as an adjunct in those particular cases. It also has a strong potential for superiority during the placement of S2 Alar-iliac screws (S2A-I). Bederman et al. point out that a nearly 100% accuracy rate was achieved with 31 robot-guided S2A-I screws with free-hand palpation, although there were 6 lateral iliac protrusions >4 mm in this cohort [43]. At the author's institution, a 94% success rate for accurate placement was achieved in the first 72 robotic S2A-I screw attempts. Shilingford et al., however, conducted a retrospective review of robotic versus free-hand S2A-I and found no perceivable difference between the two techniques with regard to accuracy [48]. Shilingford et al. however integrate data from top spinal experts which could distort the data as compared to the general spine surgeon. Surgeon specific factors remain vitally important.

Although robotic-assisted spine surgery is still at its infancy, it has been shown to be effective and safe as a pedicle screw placement technique. More evidence, in terms of large prospective comparative studies, is needed to prove the superiority of robotic-assisted spine surgery over computer-assisted navigation and free-hand techniques since the available data suggests equipoise between the three techniques of pedicle cannulation. Thus, large, carefully controlled prospective studies comparing the overall accuracy and safety of robotic-assisted cannulation with the other techniques is warranted. The surgeon's training and experience should always be considered as well. It is largely established that surgeons who are conversant with all spinal instrumentation techniques are unlikely to report large differences in accuracy between the techniques.

In the same breath, again, many young surgeons have trained in programs that exclusively utilize CT-navigation, MIS, or robotic techniques and, consequently, are likely to report significant discrepancy between one of the aforementioned techniques and a true freehand technique. It is, therefore, crucial that available data on the techniques be interpreted in a cautious manner. Surgeons must identify and acknowledge their abilities and limitations with each technique so as to enhance patient safety. We predict that more surgeons will embrace this technology as it becomes more prevalent due to reduced cost of acquiring and operating surgical robotic technology.

Cost Consideration

A realistic appreciation for the cost of technology is applicable. There are several barriers to the integration of technology at the hospital, provider, and third-party level. Hospital systems are concerned about overhead expenditures with a greater focus on the immediate fiscal period. Different technologies will have different fixed and variable cost structures. Private insurance companies are concerned about the immediate cost of something only during the period in which they are to cover the patient. Long-term savings over the lifetime of a patient are generally not of immediate concern. Surgeons are focused chiefly on patient related outcomes and healing the person to the best of their ability. Meanwhile government agencies focus within a budget, a budget that disproportionately is responsible for coverage in patients over the age of 65. This triangularization of priorities can make new technology adaptation difficult.

Research is shifting to a cost conscious perspective regarding technology adaptation. For example, investigation has seen robotic technology as a viable option for a hospital health system. Conservative savings were estimated at $608,546 for a year period of integration of robotic technology to active spine surgery practice at an academic center performing just over five-hundred and fifty fusions per year [25]. Dea et al. noted that the computer assisted spinal surgery became cost effective at institutions where more than 254 instrumented spinal procedures were performed per year due to reduced re-operation rates [49]. Minimally invasive transforaminal interbody fusions reduced mean hospital cost by $1758, indirect cost by $8474, and two-year societal cost by $9295 as compared to open TLIFs [50]. Technology in spine surgery is outlined in Table 9.1.

Table 9.1 Technology in spine surgery

Technology	Benefits	Risk	Opportunity
Pedicle screw fixation	Biomechanical advantage	Can result in technical challenges for placement Potential spinal cord and nerve root risk	Three-column control of the spine for deformity correction
Neuromonitoring	Real-time feedback of spinal cord, thecal sac, and nerve roots	Need for development of neuromonitoring protocol and neuromonitoring team Proper integration of data by surgeon	Allows for intra-operative adjustments and responses to changes in data
Minimally invasive spine techniques	Possibility to decrease soft tissue damage	Steep-learning curve Possible increased operative time Concern about fusion	Possible decreased pain, length of stay, infection, and cost Patient optics
Intra-operative CT imaging	Allows for very detailed intraoperative imaging capabilities	Significant sunken cost Radiation exposure Cumbersome size Additional operative time	Confirmation of pedicle screw placement Allows for Intraoperative adjustments and analysis
Intraoperative CT navigation	Allows for direct visualization during placement of pedicle screws	Can develop reliance on technology Significant sunken cost Radiation exposure	Increased confidence in placement of pedicle screws
Robotic spine technology	Possibility of increased pedicle screw placement accuracy Significant opportunities for intraoperative planning with software	Can develop reliance on technology Emerging technology Loss of surgeon control Significant sunken cost Surgeon and staff learning curve	Integration of technology as an aide in specifically challenging pedicle screw anatomy or minimally invasive techniques May be coupled with CT navigation

Conclusion

The twenty-first century brought with it drastic technological advances in spine surgery, resulting in useful tools for surgeons to use in addressing spinal disorders. Improvements in spine instrumentation, imaging capabilities, neuromonitoring, osteotomy and fusion techniques, antifibrinolytic therapies, and minimally invasive techniques have dramatically altered the way surgeons go about their business, thereby improving their ability to fix increasingly complex spinal conditions in an effective and safe manner. It is important that these technologies do not replace surgical principles, such as careful surgical planning, thorough understanding of pathoanatomy, and intense attention to detail during surgery, strict indications, and always preceding with a high degree of caution and alertness. All the technological tools discussed should be regarded as mere tools that aid the surgeon to achieve highest safety within the operating room and should not be taken to enhance safety independently.

References

1. Diffusion of Innovation Theory. Available at http://sphweb.bumc.bu.edu/otlt/MPH-Modules/SB/BehavioralChangeTheories/BehavioralChangeTheories4.html. Accessed 23 Oct 2018.
2. Menger RP, Connor DE, Thakur JD, et al. A comparison of lumboperitoneal and ventriculoperitoneal shunting for idiopathic intracranial hypertension: an analysis of economic impact and complications using the Nationwide Inpatient Sample. Neurosurg Focus. 2014;37:E4.
3. Harrington PR. Treatment of scoliosis. Correction and internal fixation by spine instrumentation. J Bone Joint Surg Am. 1962;44-A:591–610.
4. Moe JH, Kharrat K, Winter RB, et al. Harrington instrumentation without fusion plus external orthotic support for the treatment of difficult curvature problems in young children. Clin Orthop. 1984;1(185):35–45.
5. Knoeller SM, Seifried C. Historical perspective: history of spinal surgery. Spine. 2000;25:2838–43.
6. Hasler CC. A brief overview of 100 years of history of surgical treatment for adolescent idiopathic scoliosis. J Child Orthop. 2013;7:57–62.
7. Harrington PR, Tullos HS. Reduction of severe spondylolisthesis in children. South Med J. 1969;62:1–7.

8. Roy-Camille R, Roy-Camille M, Demeulenaere C. Osteosynthesis of dorsal, lumbar, and lumbosacral spine with metallic plates screwed into vertebral pedicles and articular apophyses. Presse Med. 1970;78:1447–8.
9. Schwab F, Blondel B, Chay E, et al. The comprehensive anatomical spinal osteotomy classification. Neurosurgery. 2015;76:S33–41.
10. Lenke LG, Sides BA, Koester LA, et al. Vertebral column resection for the treatment of severe spinal deformity. Clin Orthop. 2010;468:687–99.
11. Saifi C, Laratta JL, Petridis P, et al. Vertebral column resection for rigid spinal deformity. Glob Spine J. 2017;7:280–90.
12. Gum JL, Carreon LY, Buchowski JM, et al. Utilization trends of pedicle subtraction osteotomies compared to posterior spinal fusion for deformity: a national database analysis between 2008–2011. Scoliosis Spinal Disord. 11. Epub ahead of print August 24, 2016. https://doi.org/10.1186/s13013-016-0081-z.
13. Chan P, Andras LM, Nielsen E, et al. Comparison of Ponte osteotomies and 3-column osteotomies in the treatment of congenital spinal deformity. J Pediatr Orthop. Epub ahead of print August 2017. https://doi.org/10.1097/BPO.0000000000001057.
14. Laratta JL, Ha A, Shillingford JN, et al. Neuromonitoring in spinal deformity surgery: a multimodality approach. Glob Spine J. 2018;8:68–77.
15. Vauzelle C, Stagnara P, Jouvinroux P. Functional monitoring of spinal cord activity during spinal surgery. Clin Orthop. 1973;93:173–8.
16. Nuwer MR, Dawson EG, Carlson LG, et al. Somatosensory evoked potential spinal cord monitoring reduces neurologic deficits after scoliosis surgery: results of a large multicenter survey. Electroencephalogr Clin Neurophysiol. 1995;96:6–11.
17. Gunnarsson T, Krassioukov AV, Sarjeant R, et al. Real-time continuous intraoperative electromyographic and somatosensory evoked potential recordings in spinal surgery: correlation of clinical and electrophysiologic findings in a prospective, consecutive series of 213 cases. Spine. 2004;29:677–84.
18. Schwartz DM, Auerbach JD, Dormans JP, et al. Neurophysiological detection of impending spinal cord injury during scoliosis surgery. J Bone Joint Surg Am. 2007;89:2440–9.
19. Fehlings MG, Brodke DS, Norvell DC, et al. The evidence for intraoperative neurophysiological monitoring in spine surgery: does it make a difference? Spine. 2010;35:S37–46.
20. Lesser RP, Raudzens P, Lüders H, et al. Postoperative neurological deficits may occur despite unchanged intraoperative somatosensory evoked potentials. Ann Neurol. 1986;19:22–5.
21. Ben-David B, Haller G, Taylor P. Anterior spinal fusion complicated by paraplegia. A case report of a false-negative somatosensory-evoked potential. Spine. 1987;12:536–9.
22. Minahan RE, Sepkuty JP, Lesser RP, et al. Anterior spinal cord injury with preserved neurogenic "motor" evoked potentials. Clin Neurophysiol. 2001;112:1442–50.

23. Sutter M, Eggspuehler A, Grob D, et al. The diagnostic value of multi-modal intraoperative monitoring (MIOM) during spine surgery: a prospective study of 1,017 patients. Eur Spine J. 2007;16(Suppl 2):S162–70.

24. Menger R, Hefner MI, Savardekar AR, et al. Minimally invasive spine surgery in the pediatric and adolescent population: a case series. Surg Neurol Int. 2018;9:116.

25. Menger RP, Savardekar AR, Farokhi F, et al. A cost-effectiveness analysis of the integration of robotic spine technology in spine surgery. Neurospine. 2018;15:216–24.

26. Adogwa O, Parker SL, Bydon A, et al. Comparative effectiveness of minimally invasive versus open transforaminal lumbar interbody fusion: 2-year assessment of narcotic use, return to work, disability, and quality of life. J Spinal Disord Tech. 2011;24:479–84.

27. Tian N-F, Wu Y-S, Zhang X-L, et al. Minimally invasive versus open transforaminal lumbar interbody fusion: a meta-analysis based on the current evidence. Eur Spine J. 2013;22:1741–9.

28. Seng C, Siddiqui MA, Wong KPL, et al. Five-year outcomes of minimally invasive versus open transforaminal lumbar interbody fusion: a matched-pair comparison study. Spine. 2013;38:2049–55.

29. Lee KH, Yue WM, Yeo W, et al. Clinical and radiological outcomes of open versus minimally invasive transforaminal lumbar interbody fusion. Eur Spine J. 2012;21:2265–70.

30. Goldstein CL, Macwan K, Sundararajan K, et al. Perioperative outcomes and adverse events of minimally invasive versus open posterior lumbar fusion: meta-analysis and systematic review. J Neurosurg Spine. 2016;24:416–27.

31. Neal CJ, Rosner MK. Resident learning curve for minimal-access transforaminal lumbar interbody fusion in a military training program. Neurosurg Focus. 2010;28:E21.

32. Lehman RA, Lenke LG, Keeler KA, et al. Computed tomography evaluation of pedicle screws placed in the pediatric deformed spine over an 8-year period. Spine. 2007;32:2679–84.

33. Parker SL, McGirt MJ, Farber SH, et al. Accuracy of free-hand pedicle screws in the thoracic and lumbar spine: analysis of 6816 consecutive screws. Neurosurgery. 2011;68:170–8; discussion 178.

34. Bourgeois AC, Faulkner AR, Pasciak AS, et al. The evolution of image-guided lumbosacral spine surgery. Ann Transl Med. 2015;3:69.

35. Berlemann U, Heini P, Müller U, et al. Reliability of pedicle screw assessment utilizing plain radiographs versus CT reconstruction. Eur Spine J. 1997;6:406–10.

36. Mason A, Paulsen R, Babuska JM, et al. The accuracy of pedicle screw placement using intraoperative image guidance systems. J Neurosurg Spine. 2014;20:196–203.

37. Tian NF, Huang QS, Zhou P, Zhou Y, Wu R, Lou YXH. Pedicle screw insertion accuracy with different assisted methods: a systematic review and meta-analysis of comparative studies. Eur Spine J. 2011;20:846–59.

38. Kantelhardt SR, Martinez R, Baerwinkel S, et al. Perioperative course and accuracy of screw positioning in conventional, open robotic-guided and percutaneous robotic-guided, pedicle screw placement. Eur Spine J. 2011;20:860–8.

39. Schatlo B, Molliqaj G, Cuvinciuc V, et al. Safety and accuracy of robot-assisted versus fluoroscopy-guided pedicle screw insertion for degenerative diseases of the lumbar spine: a matched cohort comparison. J Neurosurg Spine. 2014;20:636–43.

40. Molliqaj G, Schatlo B, Alaid A, et al. Accuracy of robot-guided versus freehand fluoroscopy-assisted pedicle screw insertion in thoracolumbar spinal surgery. Neurosurg Focus. 2017;42:E14.

41. Joseph JR, Smith BW, Liu X, et al. Current applications of robotics in spine surgery: a systematic review of the literature. Neurosurg Focus. 2017;42:E2.

42. Overley SC, Cho SK, Mehta AI, et al. Navigation and robotics in spinal surgery: where are we now? Neurosurgery. 2017;80:S86–99.

43. Bederman SS, Hahn P, Colin V, et al. Robotic guidance for S2-alar-iliac screws in spinal deformity correction. Clin Spine Surg. 2017;30:E49–53.

44. Gao S, Lv Z, Fang H. Robot-assisted and conventional freehand pedicle screw placement: a systematic review and meta-analysis of randomized controlled trials. Eur Spine J. 2018;27:921–30.

45. Yu L, Chen X, Margalit A, et al. Robot-assisted vs freehand pedicle screw fixation in spine surgery – a systematic review and a meta-analysis of comparative studies. Int J Med Robot Comput Assist Surg. 2018;14:e1892.

46. Kim H-J, Kang K-T, Chun H-J, et al. Comparative study of 1-year clinical and radiological outcomes using robot-assisted pedicle screw fixation and freehand technique in posterior lumbar interbody fusion: a prospective, randomized controlled trial. Int J Med Robot Comput Assist Surg. 2018;14:e1917.

47. Park SM, Kim HJ, Lee SY, et al. Radiographic and clinical outcomes of robot-assisted posterior pedicle screw fixation: two-year results from a randomized controlled trial. Yonsei Med J. 2018;59:438–44.

48. Shillingford JN, Laratta JL, Park PJ, et al. Human versus robot: a propensity-matched analysis of the accuracy of free hand versus robotic guidance for placement of S2 alar-iliac (S2AI) screws. Spine. 2018;43:E1297–304.

49. Dea N, Fisher CG, Batke J, et al. Economic evaluation comparing intraoperative cone beam CT-based navigation and conventional fluoroscopy for the placement of spinal pedicle screws: a patient-level data cost-effectiveness analysis. Spine J. 2016;16:23–31.

50. Parker SL, Mendenhall SK, Shau DN, et al. Minimally invasive versus open transforaminal lumbar interbody fusion for degenerative spondylolisthesis: comparative effectiveness and cost-utility analysis. World Neurosurg. 2014;82:230–8.

51. Vitale MG, Skaggs DL, Pace GI, et al. Best practices in intraoperative neuromonitoring in spine deformity surgery: development of an intraoperative checklist to optimize response. Spine Deform. 2014;2(5):333–9.

Index

Printed in the United States
By Bookmasters